MW00583607

PLANTFED MAMA'S
HOLISTIC GUIDE TO A
Vegan Pregnancy

Candy Marx, MH, HHP

AN ETHICAL BOOK
First published in 2019 by
Ethical Press
AUSTRALIA | USA

Text copyright © Candice Marx and Ethical Press
Design © Ethical Press
Photography © Candice Marx and Ethical Press
Cover Photo Tania Niwa
Graphic Design Richell Balansag
Edited by Ethical Press
Props and Food Styling Candice Marx
Food preparation Candice Marx

The moral right of the author has been asserted.

All rights reserved. No part of this book may be reproduced, copied or transmitted by any person or entity in any form or means, digital, electronic or mechanical, including photocopying, scanning or recording, without prior permission in writing and signed by the publisher.

We advise that the information in this book is for general informational purposes only and does not negate the personal responsibility of the reader for their own health and safety. It is recommended to seek tailored professional advice from a healthcare practitioner or medical professional. The publishers and their employees, agents, and authors are not liable for injuries or damage to any person as a result of reading and following the information in this book.

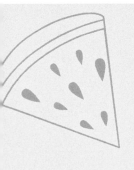

"WE ARE RAISING THE NEXT
GENERATION OF LEADERS AND
CHANGEMAKERS. IT'S ESSENTIAL THAT
OUR CHILDREN ARE COMPASSIONATE,
HEALTHY AND WELL-LOVED."

CM

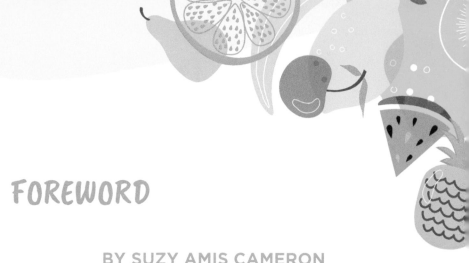

FOREWORD

BY SUZY AMIS CAMERON

Babies. And pregnant mamas. I've got a thing about them. There's nothing more exciting than a new little person coming into this world! I remember so vividly being pregnant – and how I felt the responsibility (and joy!) of taking care of this itty-bitty life growing inside me. You want so much to do everything right.

Looking back 28 years, when I gave birth to my first baby, Jasper, it seems like we were in the dark ages of nutritional science around plant-based eating. I'm pretty sure that plant-based nutritionists didn't even exist. Now, as an expectant *grandmother* to my son and daughter-in-law's first baby, I am thrilled to learn about Candy's incredible and encouraging resource, *Plantfed Mama's Holistic Guide to a Vegan Pregnancy.*

Our science and knowledge have come so far, and *Plantfed Mama* Candy breaks it down for us. She shares how expectant mothers – and those who support them! – can now make sure they're getting all of the vitamins and minerals they need, understand wholefoods and the lifeforce energy in it, and take advantage of good carbs, fats, and proteins. She also addresses pregnancy-specific issues with foods that can help certain challenges, such as morning sickness, cramps and edema, gestational diabetes, and so much more.

Swollen feet? Tummy issues? Herbal remedies for labor? Exhaustion? *Plantfed Mama* is here!

As Candy is a nutritionist and herbalist, this book is the ideal midwife-on-the-shelf to support a plant-based diet during pregnancy and beyond. And let's not forget the most important thing: feeding the mama! OMG the recipes! Scrumptiously delicious and colorful – smoothies, wraps, tortillas, fritters, rolls, burgers, pastas, soups, noodles, and (wait for it): "nicecream."

Plantfed Mama is an incredible example of the amazing power of mothers helping mothers. When I was pregnant, I turned to sisters, experienced mother friends, and books that helped me with middle-of-the-night mystery rashes, questionable fevers, and nursing dilemmas. We're connected as mothers and daughters, in this extraordinary group of fierce, vulnerable women, or mother bears. And now with Candy's help, we can support ourselves and the ripe, gorgeous *Plantfed Mamas* in our lives. I can't wait to give this book out to every new mom I know, now, and in the years to come.

Suzy Amis Cameron

(Author, Film Producer, Conservationist, Founder of MUSE School CA, Vegan Wife & Mama)

www.suzyamiscameron.com

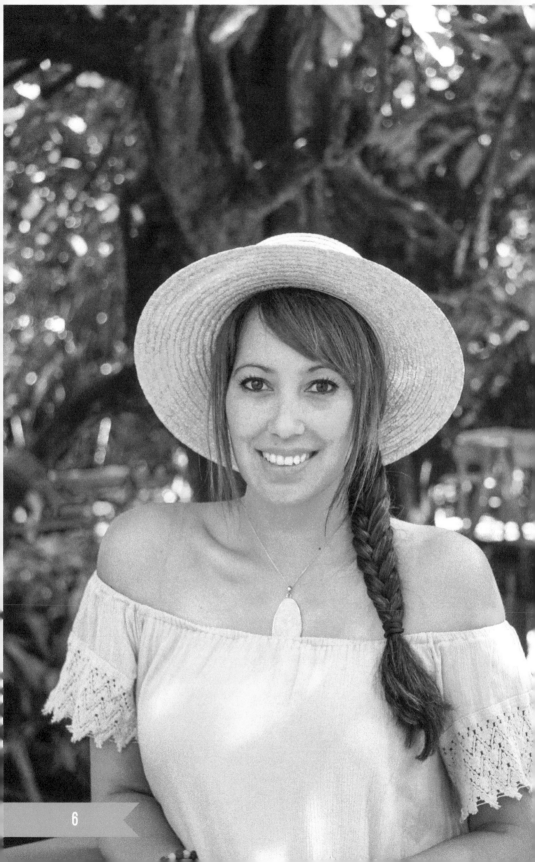

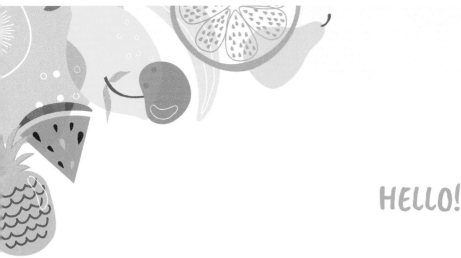

HELLO!

Hey! I'm Candy, and I'm a registered Plant-based Nutritionist and registered Master Herbalist. Some of you might know me as Plantfed Mama, my popular Instagram account, where I share nutritious plant-based recipes, and nutritional, holistic, and spiritual advice, or from my podcast, Plantfed Soul. I currently live on Sydney's Northern Beaches, with my healthy vegan family.

I grew up on a small self-sustained farm in Hawkes Bay, New Zealand, where my lifestyle was simple. We lived mostly off the land, and our gigantic football-field-sized garden was fun to maintain. We had twelve different varieties of blooming heritage fruit trees, which is where we grabbed our daily snacks. We climbed trees, built forts, and our phone number only consisted of three digits. The ocean was a five-minute drive away, where we would spend entire days. I guess that is why I have always had a love for fresh food, the outdoors, and well, for animals.

I was a kid when I made the connection between our dogs and our pigs. Our pigs ran to us when called, they loved a bum scratch, and they even kicked their back leg when we rubbed their bellies. After making that connection, it was evident to me that I had to stop eating animals. This was at a time when vegetarians didn't really exist in my known world, and it was still considered dangerous and unhealthy to give up meat. I was lucky enough to be surrounded by a plethora of fresh and organic produce, and this is pretty much where I began my love for plant-based wholefoods.

I was a vegetarian for around fifteen years, and I made the transition to vegan and plant-based in 2012.

I'm a huge supporter of my local grower's markets, where I buy all of my weekly produce. I love supporting small businesses, and I always make an effort to go — rain, hail, or shine. Whatever I can't buy from the markets, I source from the local health shop and bulk foods store. It's also incredibly important to me to use as little plastic as possible and filling up jars or paper bags at the bulk foods store eliminates single-use plastic bags. Using mesh produce bags instead of plastic produce bags is also a good swap. Not only is plastic an environmental problem, but toxins can leach into many of the foods wrapped and packaged in plastic.

I am the mama of two gorgeous souls: my daughter, Keilana, and my son, Kaimana. I was 100% plant-based and vegan while carrying Kaimana, and I was primarily plant-based while carrying Keilana. Both of my children were healthy at birth and weighed over 7.5 pounds. I mention this because when people found out that I was having a vegan pregnancy while carrying Kaimana, the majority assumed that he would be a 'small baby.' Funnily enough, at three-months-old, Kaimana was wearing six-to-twelve-month-old clothing! And at ten-weeks, he was almost the same size as his six-month-old cousin. We're definitely breaking the stigma of vegans being small, unhealthy, and weak!

Until recently, a baby that weighed over 7.5 pounds was considered big, and the size of these babies was typically blamed on mama's poor diet, excessive weight gain, and/or gestational diabetes. However, there is a massive difference between 'sumo babies' and babies who are larger than average.

I can assure you that I didn't put on excessive weight during either of my pregnancies, nor did I have gestational diabetes. Researchers have noticed a trend in larger babies, which they say could be due to our increasing good health. As a society, we no longer smoke cigarettes as much as we used to, we're generally eating better, and we're more aware of the toxins in our environment. The list goes on. So, while 'big babies' can be because mama overate, or genetics, it can also be because mama sufficiency fuelled her body and baby. I'm also a huge believer that a healthy body will create a baby that mama can safely birth.

Back in 2008, when I was pregnant with my daughter, I wasn't in a position to question my doctor's orders. I didn't know enough about nutrition to be confident in a vegan or vegetarian pregnancy, so I added some seafood back to my diet, while primarily eating fruit and vegetables. I now know exactly what to eat and how to thrive during a vegan pregnancy. I've met so many vegan women who want to continue being vegan during their pregnancies, but there is a lack of information and pressure from others who don't understand how healthy a plant-based lifestyle can be. That is why I wrote this book.

During my second pregnancy, I had my blood and urine tested. I made sure not to tell my doctor that I was 100% plant-based and had been for years, because, in my experience health practitioners even holistic practitioners, have pre-judged and assumed that eating meat was necessary. When I went back for the results, my doctor was speechless because my results were "too healthy." Yes, my doctor joked and literally said that! I tested almost perfectly in just about everything: vitamin count, mineral count, and blood cell count. My protein, lipid and glucose levels were nearly perfect. My urine tested a pH of 8, and I only tested low in the things that should be low, like uric acid, urate, and cholesterol. In case you're wondering, our bodies naturally produce cholesterol and it's essential for our bodies to produce vitamin D. Contrary to popular belief, vitamin D is actually a hormone. I had the same tests done at twenty-eight-weeks pregnant, and my results were again, almost perfect.

One thing that stayed with me from my pregnancies was how much my intuition grew. I have been spiritual for most of my life, so that side has also been part of me, but I didn't know just how much pregnancy strengthens it. When I was carrying Keilana, I knew things that I shouldn't have known, and if someone was to tell me differently, I knew in every bone of my body that I was right. While carrying Kaimana, my intuition strengthened even more. I will go into more detail about this in Chapter 18.

I wrote most of this book while I was pregnant with Kaimana. It was incredibly important to me to be going through a vegan pregnancy while writing a book about it. The experience enabled me to add information that I wouldn't have even thought about adding, had I not been going through it myself. I also perfected most of the recipes in this book and took every photo during my third trimester, which was definitely a challenge, so I hope you like them!

I love science, and I love spirituality, and it's important for me to bridge that gap. Once I experienced the incredible health benefits of a wholefoods plant-based diet, I was determined to study plants from a medicinal and nutritional side. Which is why I studied a double diploma, in Master Herbalism and Human Nutrition. I also wanted to combine my scientific knowledge with my spiritual knowledge, thus moving towards Holistic Health. It's also important to me to continue learning. New discoveries are made every day, and degrees and diplomas only mean so much if we don't continue learning after we've finished our studies. It's crucial that we keep an eye on new research, clinical trials, and nutritional studies.

An example of why it's crucial to continue learning is back when I was still studying Herbalism. I tried everything to help my daughter who wasn't feeling well, so I took her to see a Naturopath/ Herbalist. During the consultation, the Naturopath realized that we were a vegan family and the diagnosis became about that. In her opinion, my daughter was sick because we were vegan and not getting enough vitamins and minerals in our diet, even though I had explained that we eat wholefoods and are very conscious of our nutrient intake. She prescribed B12, zinc, an herbal tincture, and prescription-only-probiotics.

From my own training, prescribing anyone supplements without testing for deficiencies is dangerous. The B12 supplement also contained dairy-derived lactose. It turned out that my daughter had tonsillitis, and I diagnosed her because I caught it the week after. This also explained why it took a couple of weeks for my daughter to recover. My point here is that if practitioners aren't continuing to learn, assumptions and mistakes are made. This applies to all disciplines including Western medicine, Eastern medicine, and Holistic Health.

Throughout your pregnancy, it's super crucial to listen to yourself, your intuition, and your body. If you're tired, rest. If you're hungry, eat. If anyone suggests something that doesn't feel right to you, don't do it. Always speak up, especially in the delivery room. Some midwives and OB/GYNs have been known to stick to 'a schedule', which puts unnecessary pressure on mama, but you got this. Listen to yourself and speak up when you need to. It's your time, and if there is anything that you want or anything that you don't want, say so. It isn't rude to ask!

If you're wondering what an Herbalist is, an Herbalist is an alternative and holistic health practitioner (H.H.P) who has studied plant science intended for medicinal purposes, as well as human anatomy, Ayurveda, herbal medicine, and nutrition. Herbalists treat the body holistically: physically, mentally and spiritually, and use plants medicinally to improve health, promote healing, and prevent and treat illness. Herbal medicine, also called herbalism, botanical medicine, or phytomedicine, has been used for thousands of years.

I invited Suzy Amis Cameron to write the foreword and Paul de Gelder to write the afterword for this book because I wanted to include both perspectives – female and male. Both Suzy and Paul come from completely different parts of the world, yet like me, they share a love of veganism, conservation, and wellness.

I made it my mission to offer as much information as I could, because to me, the right information empowers! If you're new to veganism or plant-based eating, or if you've been vegan for a while, or even if you aren't vegan, you'll learn a lot from this book. Take it one step at a time and refer back whenever you need to.

I don't have to tell you that a vegan diet is better for animals, and for the environment, but I hope that by reading this book, you'll feel empowered in your decision to have a vegan pregnancy. I hope you'll feel confident in your food choices and knowing that you're getting enough nutrients into yours and baby's diet.

Candy xxxx

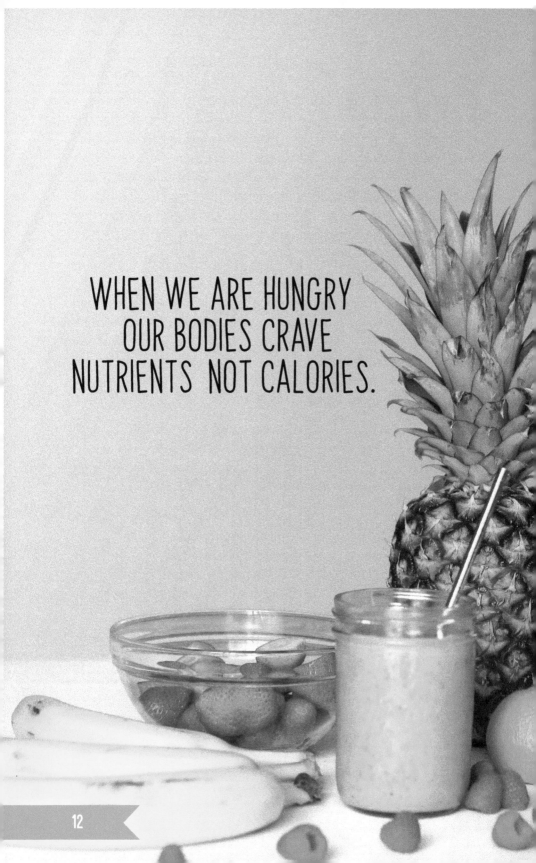

WHEN WE ARE HUNGRY
OUR BODIES CRAVE
NUTRIENTS NOT CALORIES.

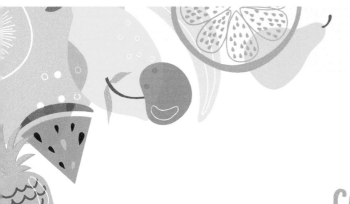

CONTENTS

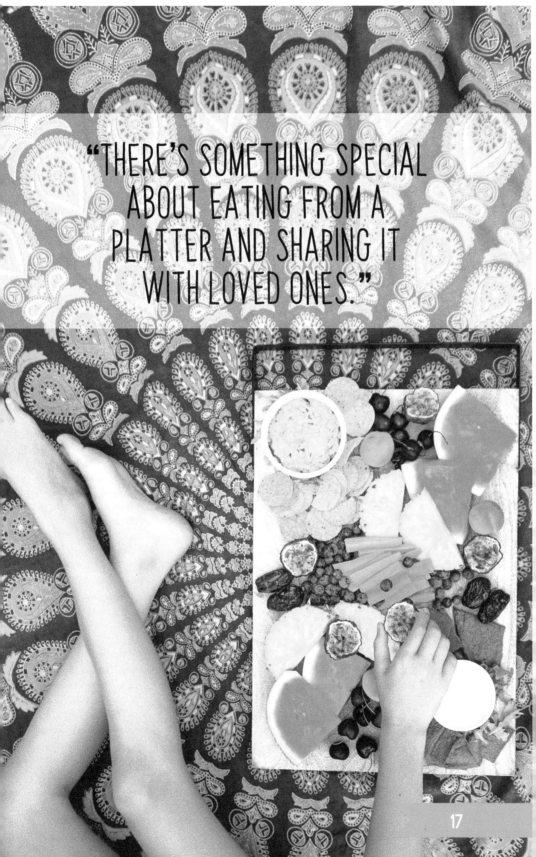

"THERE'S SOMETHING SPECIAL ABOUT EATING FROM A PLATTER AND SHARING IT WITH LOVED ONES."

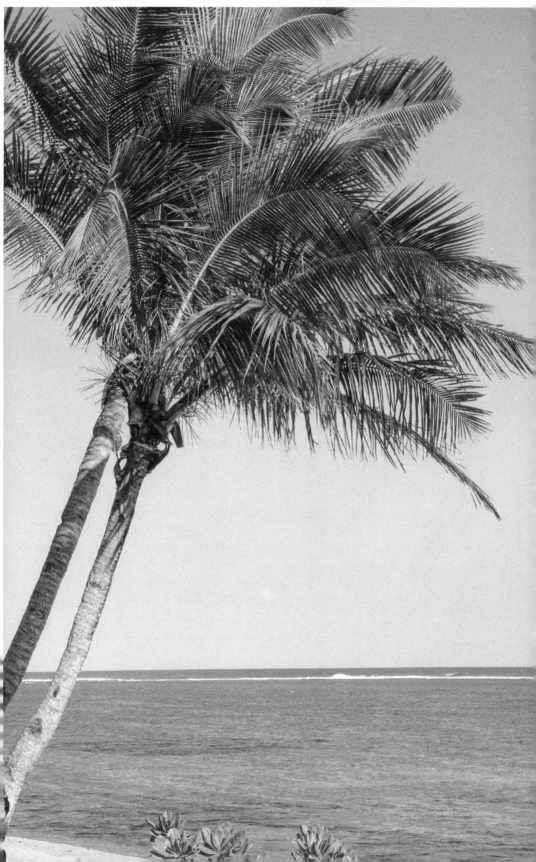

CHAPTER 1

What I Eat and My Kitchen Staples

I'm often asked how much I spend per week on food, or if I use crazy, hard-to-source ingredients. While I'm totally practical in the kitchen and buy what is available to me, I can't put a price on my or my family's health. I will always opt to buy better quality food over purchasing new gadgets or accessories. Considering we buy all organic ingredients, the reality is that my family and I spend about AU$150 per week at our local grower's market, where we buy all of our fresh produce. We also spend about AU$100 or so at our local health shop, and about AU$50 per fortnight at our local bulk foods store.

Over the years, especially when I first began eating high-raw, I was given several 'raw cookbooks', and I pretty much knew straight away whether I'd use the recipes in them or not. I've never been someone who makes recipes that use a whole heap of ingredients, with hard-to-source ingredients, or that expect us to be in the kitchen for hours at a time. I joke a lot and call myself a 'lazy cook,' but the reality is, I'm practical, as you will see from the recipes in this book. And as it turns out 'practical food' is healthy food; food that is closest to its original source, less processed, and not over-cooked.

I eat a lot of fruit. Fruit and filtered water are the largest staples in my diet, followed by vegetables. After vegetables, I eat smaller amounts of legumes, nuts, and some seeds. Grains are at the top of my food pyramid (meaning that I eat grains the least), along with general herbs and spices.

I always start my day with fruit, either a few pieces of fruit, a smoothie, or a smoothie bowl. Fruit energizes the body with glucose (the body's main fuel source) which is the perfect way to start the day. If you like lemon tea (lemon steeped in hot water) start with that, then eat fruit about twenty minutes after.

When we sleep our bodies are in healing, recuperation, and detox mode. Upon awakening, our bodies continue to be in detox mode, so eating fruit ensures the body's energy is used for detox rather than digesting heavy foods. Fruit softly wakes up the digestive system and fiber helps to clean the colon. Many tend to reach for coffee upon waking, which delivers a massive jolt to the central nervous system and the digestive system. In fact, fruit is the perfect coffee replacer; it's gentle on the entire body, and due to the natural sugars which convert into glucose, it helps fuel the body, including the brain. Fruit delivers true energy that sustains the body over a longer period of time.

Smoothie bowls keep me full and satisfied for hours, so if that is how I start, I usually just snack on more fruit, nuts, or rice paper rolls throughout the rest of the day. If I'm extra hungry, I'll bake sweet potato wedges and serve them with guacamole and salad, or make a chickpea sun bowl (recipes at the back of the book). During pregnancy, mainly after five months in, I was noticeably hungrier, so I made extra food at dinnertime and ate the leftovers for lunch the next day. It's really not necessary to 'eat for two' especially in the earlier months, but it is crucial to keep up a regular flow of nutrients.

Before pregnancy, I fasted intermittently. I ate dinner at around 7pm and breakfast between 11am - 12pm. This came naturally to me because I was never hungry in the morning. I also prefer to do yoga on an empty stomach, so I'd always eat after my yoga practice. But during pregnancy, I ate when I was hungry, and surprisingly, not a lot changed with the size of my appetite until I reached my fifth month.

Eating several smaller snacks or meals, rather than three large meals, is ideal for that regular flow of nutrients. It's also easier on the digestive system and helps alleviate nausea. With all of the 'moving around' that's going on inside of a pregnant woman's body, larger meals and hard-to-digest foods can lead to constipation. And backed-up plumbing strains the butt which can contribute to haemorrhoids during labour. Always relieve yourself when you need to go.

My dinners are always full of fresh and/or cooked vegetables, paired with legumes and/or certain grains. I sometimes add something like corn chips or tortillas to our meals, depending on what we're having. My absolute favourite legumes are lentils and chickpeas. I love the flavours and how versatile these legumes are. I also love freshly prepared broad beans, and I eat other beans, but not as much as lentils and chickpeas. They also happen to top the list of the most nutritious legumes, and lentils are rich in prebiotics. I also love tempeh and I eat tofu every now and then.

Because a lot of soy is GMO, and because soy contains phytoestrogens, or plant-based estrogens, soy has received a bad rap. However, phytoestrogens do not act the same way as estrogen. When phytoestrogens occupy the cell, normal estrogens cannot. Phytoestrogens do not eliminate or block estrogen's effects, but they do minimize them. What a lot of people seem to forget is that meat, dairy, and eggs contain high levels of actual estrogen, which does affect the hormones. Phytoestrogens in soy do not appear to have any effect on hormone levels, but animal estrogen certainly does.

Tofu isn't as processed as many people believe. Traditional tofu is simply soaked, blended and cooked soybeans set in nigari. You can make your own tofu at home! Always purchase organic and non-GMO soy products, fermented is even better. And like many foods, don't overconsume.

I eat a handful of nuts and seeds on most days, mainly almonds, Brazil nuts, pistachios, and hemp seeds. I use cashews and macadamias in creams, cheeses, baking, and raw desserts, and chia seeds in jams. Otherwise, I don't usually eat chia; I have gone into more detail about this in Chapter 8.

Nuts, seeds, and dates can go rancid quite quickly, especially in warmer months, so store them in airtight jars in the fridge. If you use hemp oil, hemp seeds, flaxseed oil, flaxseed, or flax meal, store them in the fridge too. When it comes to purchasing herbs and spices, opt for spices that are sold in glass jars over plastic. Buying herbs and spices in glass jars not only eliminates plastic, but we also have no idea how long these foods have sat on the shelves, and glass helps to keep the herbs fresher for longer.

The only downside about using bulk food stores is that many do not keep their produce in airtight bulk bins. I found this out the hard way after purchasing a large bag of nuts that were mostly rancid. These types of foods must be stored properly, otherwise they quickly go rancid. Most rancid nuts will float when soaked in water, and they will taste and feel stale as well. Fresh dates are soft, while old dates are tough and wrinkled.

While I'm not grain-free, I avoid conventional wheat and grains. I can eat small amounts of organic sourdough bread made using wild-yeast and stoneground, unbleached flour, but my bread intake is very limited. It is also important to factor in the qualities of the flours that are used because most are bleached, have additives, preservatives, and are laden with pesticides. Much of the gluten dissipates in the fermentation process when making sourdough bread which makes it easier to digest. However, not all sourdough is created equal. True sourdough is fermented for at least twenty-four hours, and it's made with wild-yeast. This sourdough is much better to consume and can actually help build the beneficial bacteria in the gut. I avoid added yeast due to its candida-feeding properties, which I will cover further on.. Gluten is acidic and can be inflammatory, so I don't overdo it. However, if gluten upsets your gut, genetically-modified wheat is also something to consider.

While it is best to source local produce whenever possible, European wheat acts differently than standard wheat. European wheat is *soft wheat* that has less gluten which is easily broken down. Here in Australia and in the USA, we have *hard wheat*. This wheat was modified to obtain a higher yield, the grain itself is larger than soft wheat, and it contains far more gluten which is hard for the body to break down.

Some people who suffer from gluten intolerances have been known to eat Italian wheat without any issue.

If you do eat wheat products make sure to always opt for organic when you can. Conventional wheat (and fruit, vegetables and other grains) is sprayed with glycophosphate (thanks to Roundup), and unfortunately, glycophosphate (also called glyphosate) enters the rain cycle as well. Glycophosphate is linked to cancer due to the blocking of the production of an enzyme in the body called CYP. This enzyme detoxifies the body; its purpose is to get rid of the chemicals that the body cannot eliminate on its own. If these enzymes cannot be produced, then the body cannot eliminate the toxins. This can lead to a number of severe health problems, including cancer and organ damage. Glycophosphate also kills gut bacteria.

I keep brown rice and teff in the pantry. I seldomly cook brown rice though it comes in handy for curries. I also try to add teff to baking. To me, most mainstream grains are more of a filler rather than nutrient-dense foods, and these mainstream grains are acidic in nature and full of phytic acid. Some people can digest these grains a lot better than others, and while I would generally say that this comes down to gut health, it also comes down to genetics.

For example, my background is Polynesian, and my ancestors mostly ate fruit, vegetables, sweet potato (kumara), and seafood. There was very little starch in this diet, no gluten, and was basically grain-free. Whereas, my husband's English and Irish ancestors ate a lot of grains, meat, and potatoes. I see the difference between the foods that he can eat without feeling bloated and sluggish, compared to the foods that I can. I see this effect in my clients as well.

Basically, I don't feel my best after eating most grains, so I avoid conventional, non-organic grains and limit my intake. I do think it's crucial to expand on what we eat and to not just follow what our ancestors ate, but it is important to keep that in mind. By this, I mean that our ancestors ate what was available to them, however, we now live in a time where a variety of foods are more accessible to us, and we're finding out more about the science of food. Many experts talk about how healthy Asian cultures are and that they mainly eat white rice, but they forget that their ancestors have been eating rice for thousands of years. Genetics is one reason why I believe some people can tolerate grains far better than others. Personally, I feel the best after eating fruit and vegetables, so that's what I mainly eat.

Another gluten-free (pseudo) grain that I keep in my pantry is buckwheat, which is high in phytic acid, but also contains high levels of phytase. Phytase is the enzyme that we lack in our digestive tract which breaks down phytic acid.

For baking and cooking, I mostly use buckwheat flour, chickpea flour, teff flour, and tapioca or arrowroot flour. Chickpea flour and buckwheat flour are super versatile, and adding tapioca or arrowroot helps to bind them, without having to use xanthum gum or guar gum.

Sugar is sugar, but some sugars are somewhat better than others. White sugar is a refined carbohydrate that I call a toxin. It is technically classified as a drug. It is said that it takes four pancreases to process white sugar, but we only have one. White sugar stresses the pancreas, liver, and kidneys, starves the brain of oxygen, and causes tooth decay, high blood pressure, infertility, and glaucoma. If you still use sugar, ditch white sugar and use a healthier and natural alternative.

I use organic Medjool dates and date paste wherever I can. Dates are a wholefood and are full of nutrients, plus they don't sharply spike the blood sugar, thanks to their fiber content. Some brands make date sugar but the sugar doesn't dissolve. This is fine for some recipes, but not for all. For recipes that call for syrup, I use date syrup or pure maple syrup. Both are processed, but still contain minerals and are low-glycemic (low-GI). I use coconut sugar for recipes that call for powdered sugar, and if I can sweeten a recipe with a ripe banana or an apple, I opt for that.

Whenever I make anything I always make sure to 'cook with intent.' This means that I make sure to be happy when I'm cooking and put 'love energy' into the food. Our energy infuses into everything that we make, whether food, art, clothing or jewelry. If we're in a bad mood, our 'bad mood energy' transfers into the food that the people we love eat. If we're in a happy, loving mood, then our high vibes transfer into the food as well. You may be surprised by the number of people who can 'taste' when the chef is in a bad mood!

I don't really have a sweet tooth. I used to but it went away after I started eating more fruit. I do like to eat raw chocolate and use cacao every now and then. Cacao is the purest form of chocolate, and when it is roasted, it becomes cocoa. Contrary to popular belief, cacao is a poor source of caffeine, but instead contains a similar chemical called *theobromine*. While theobromine is still considered a stimulant, it is about ten times weaker than caffeine, and it does not affect the central nervous system like caffeine does. Theobromine relaxes the muscles, particularly the bronchi muscles of the lungs, thus it is used to treat coughs, asthma and other respiratory illnesses. Cacao does have medicinal effects, so treat this food like any other medicinal food and do not overconsume.

Below is an example of the staples I keep in my house.

FOOD STAPLE LIST

Fruit
Whatever fruit is in season

Vegetables
Whatever vegetables are in season

Fridge/Freezer
Frozen berries/açaí/pitaya
Coconut yogurt
Plant-milk
Chopped bananas/mango/pineapple

Nut cheese

Kitchen Appliances & Tools

High-speed blender
Stick blender
Food processor
Spiralizer
Non-stick fry pan and bakeware
Note: because of the toxins in standard non-stick cookware and bakeware, I use a ceramic PTFE-free and PFOA-free fry pan, ceramic and glass baking dishes, and ceramic PTFE-free and PFOA-free muffin trays.

Powders and Flours

Cacao
Lucuma
Mesquite
Chickpea flour
Buckwheat flour
Teff flour
Flaxmeal
Tapioca or arrowroot
Masa harina

Supplements & Natural Medicine

Chlorella and/or spirulina powder
Vitamin C powder
Echinacea
Dried Elderberries
Sea moss
Sarsaparilla
Plantfed Mama Herbal blends

Herbs, Spices & Condiments

Curry powder
Garam Masala
Turmeric powder
Ground cumin
Ground cinnamon

Ground nutmeg
Dried parsley/oregano
Dried Italian herbs
Onion powder
Garlic powder
Chamomile tea
Echinacea tea
Fresh ginger
Black pepper
Pink Himalayan salt
Cayenne (used outside of pregnancy)
Tamari sauce (low sodium, alcohol-free)
Vanilla powder/extract/beans

Legumes/Grains

Lentils
Chickpeas
Black beans
Tempeh
Tofu
Buckwheat/buckwheat noodles
Brown Basmati rice
Legume pasta

Nuts and Seeds

Almonds
Cashews
Macadamias
Pistachios and/or mixed nuts
Hemp seeds
Chia seeds (for jams)

Sweeteners

Medjool dates
Date paste/syrup
Coconut sugar
Maple syrup

Butters
Cultured nut butter
Almond butter
Peanut butter
Cacao butter

I keep BPA-free cans of chickpeas and black beans in the pantry for times when I haven't planned ahead. If you use passata or bottled tomatoes opt for glass over cans or plastic, as the acid from the tomatoes has been known to eat through the can lining and leach into the food. The same can be said for citrus juices and products.

The recipes at the end of this book don't require a whole heap of ingredients, no hard-to-source ingredients, and they're simple and easy to make. Most of all, they're all nutritious! From the kitchen of this lazy cook to yours!

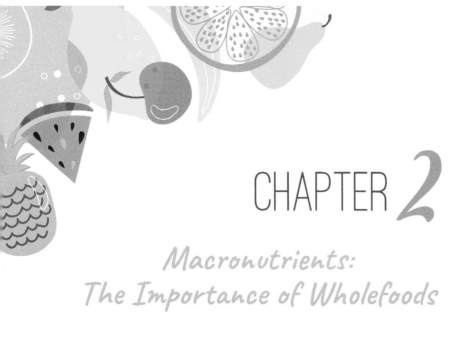

CHAPTER 2

Macronutrients: The Importance of Wholefoods

Macronutrients are nutrients that we require in higher doses, whereas, micronutrients are nutrients that we require in smaller doses. Macronutrients are carbohydrates, proteins, lipids (fats), and water. Micronutrients are vitamins and minerals, which I will cover in the next chapter.

Dietary guidelines recommend that we obtain our calories from approximately 55% carbohydrates, 30% lipids, and 15% proteins.

CARBS

Carbohydrates have had a bad reputation for a long time because people have often associated carbohydrates with weight gain, and cake, bread, pasta, and well, sugar, but carbs are found in all foods except for eggs, meat, and oils. Carbs are in fruit, vegetables, legumes and grains, and are the preferred energy source for our bodies. Carbohydrate means hydrated carbon, and is made up of carbon, hydrogen, and oxygen. When eaten, our bodies convert carbs into glucose, the primary energy source for our bodies.

Every cell in our body requires glucose. Both the brain and the central nervous system use glucose as an energy source. Some glucose is used straight away, some is stored as glycogen, and any leftover is converted into fat. Carbs only present an issue when an excess of carbs is consumed, but also, when we eat refined carbs rather than wholefood carbs.

When the body needs more energy, it converts stored glycogen back into glucose for the body to use. Our bodies are amazing, aren't they?

Now, here's why people lose weight when they give up carbs. The body burns up the glycogen which is stored in the liver and muscles. The body burns up the water that is stored with the glycogen leaving protein for the body to burn as its fuel source. The liver has to work overtime to convert protein into fuel. However, it doesn't last long, and our bodies do not like converting protein into energy due to its other vital functions. Essentially, when people give up carbs, they are predominantly losing water weight around the muscle, not necessarily losing fat.

PROTEIN

Proteins are likewise made up of carbon, hydrogen, and oxygen, but also contain nitrogen. Each protein is made up of amino acids that are linked together like beads in a necklace. We use about twenty different kinds of amino acids and arrange them into thousands of proteins.

Each amino acid is organ specific, meaning that the skin needs a different protein than the lungs and the heart. Some uses for proteins are growth, repair, and to control fluids, electrolytes, and acid-base balance in the body.

Eleven amino acids are made within the body, making these proteins non-essential. The other nine cannot be made within the body and therefore must be eaten. From the eleven non-essential amino acids, six are 'conditionally non-essential' meaning that in some people, they are usually not essential, except in times of illness and stress.

You may have heard that plant-sourced proteins are not complete proteins because they do not contain all of the essential amino acids.

This has led to many people 'food combining' grains with legumes to create complete proteins.

However, I will note that legumes, nuts, and grains do contain all of the essential amino acids, they just contain lower amounts of *lysine* and *methionine* compared to meat. Legumes are a poor source of the amino acid, methionine, and grains have higher levels. On the other hand, grains are a poor source of the amino acid, lysine, but legumes have adequate levels. This is why plants have been wrongly called 'incomplete sources of protein.' Teff, soy, quinoa, hemp seeds, chia seeds, and buckwheat in particular, are excellent sources of all amino acids.

It is also important to note that we only require low levels of methionine and lysine. Too much lysine and methionine do come with ill-effects. However, too much of anything including all of the amino acids, is a bad thing, and plants give us smaller amounts of methionine and lysine for a reason. I like to think of it as 'plants give us exactly what we need.'

While protein deficiencies are only common in developing countries, excess protein in the West is more common. When there is excess protein, the amino acids that make up the protein molecule are deaminated, which means, the nitrogen-containing amine group is separated. Deamination produces ammonia, which the cells release into the bloodstream, and the liver then takes up. The liver converts the ammonia into urea and releases it into the blood to be filtered out by the kidneys and excreted. This means that the liver and kidneys are constantly over-working trying to get rid of the ammonia, and if the liver or kidneys are already compromised, then the ammonia stays in the body and builds up. High levels of protein also inhibit nutrient absorption, such as calcium, magnesium and B-complex vitamins. You've probably been asked, "Where do you get your protein?" As you can see, plant-based eating poses minimal risk of protein deficiency, but too much protein can definitely cause harm.

Animals get their protein from the same source as us – plants! The only reason herbivore animals have protein in their bodies is because they eat plants.

LIPIDS (FATS)

Our bodies need fat and eating healthy fats should be part of every meal. Fats help keep the skin and hair healthy, and provide essential fatty acids, Omega-6 (LA or Linoleic Acid) and Omega-3 (ALA or Alpha-Linoleic Acid), which assist in the absorption of fat-soluble vitamins A, D, E, and K.

Triglycerides include monounsaturated and polyunsaturated fats and are known as *good fats*. These fats supply energy, protect against extremes and shock, and help our bodies use carbs and proteins efficiently. I include at least one good fat with every meal because the fat helps nutrients to be better absorbed. When bound to good fats, the nutrients have a higher chance of making it through the stomach and the liver, without being absorbed prematurely. Then it can be absorbed through the small intestine and transferred into the blood. My favourite sources of monounsaturated and polyunsaturated fats come from avocados, nuts, and hemp seeds.

Two types of polyunsaturated fats are Omega-3 and Omega-6. These are considered essential fatty acids because they cannot be synthesized within the body and must come from our food. It's fairly easy to eat adequate amounts of Omega-6 as it is in most vegetable oils, seeds, and nuts. But because Omega-6 is found in most vegetable oils, it is therefore found in most processed foods. In fact, it is estimated that we eat about twenty times more Omega-6 than Omega-3, so acquiring the right balance is vital.

The desired ratio of Omega-3 to Omega-6 is roughly 1:5 to 1:10. These fatty acids compete for the same enzymes; therefore, they compete for absorption, and excess in one can inhibit the absorption of the other. Omega-6 is also inflammatory, and too many Omega-6s are more detrimental than helpful.

A healthy wholefoods diet is nature's way of protecting us from eating too many of one type. Our Omega-3 and Omega-6 intake will balance itself out if we eat properly.

There are several different types of Omega-3s, and in my experience, this fatty acid is the nutrient that stumps most vegans. Alpha-linolenic acid (ALA) is a short-chain Omega-3 that contains eighteen carbon atoms, and is found in plants such as hemp seeds, chia seeds, walnuts, flaxseeds, and legumes. However, our bodies must convert ALA into long-chain Omega-3s, Docosahexaenoic acid or DHA which contains twenty carbon atoms, and Eicosapentaenoic acid or EPA which contains twenty-two carbon atoms. These are the long-chain Omega-3s found in oily fish which are crucial for the immune system and cardiovascular protection.

Like us, fish also obtain their Omega-3s from plants which is the only reason why they contain Omega-3s to begin with.

On a plant-based diet, it's crucial to consume decent amounts of Omega-3s (ALA) in order to convert it into EPA and DHA. This also means that we should lower our Omega-6s (LA) intake, especially processed Omega-6s, to allow more Omega-3s to covert.

Saturated fats, trans-fats and added cholesterol are known as bad fats; however, cholesterol is part lipid and part protein. This is why different types of cholesterol are called *lipoproteins*. While it is impossible to get every nutritionist, dietician, or scientist to agree, some say that all saturated fats are bad because they are more readily stored as fat in the body, which leads to raised levels of bad cholesterol (Low-Density Lipoprotein; LDL). Saturated fats are also linked to insulin resistance, which is the cause of type-2 Diabetes. The fat inside the muscle fibers interferes with insulin signalling. The body has to keep pumping insulin to try and force it into the muscles. The blood sugar spikes because it can't enter into the cells, where 85% of the blood sugar would typically be used. The term used to describe the effects of saturated fat is called *lipotoxicity*.

Coconut oil is a popular oil to cook with because of its nutritional properties, high smoke point, and flavour. Although it is high in saturated fats, and low in monounsaturated and polyunsaturated fats, the saturated fats are mainly from lauric acid. This is a saturated fat that is believed to act differently than other saturated fats, by increasing good cholesterol (HDL). However, some studies have shown that coconut oil may also increase bad cholesterol (LDL) too. I will admit that on occasion I use coconut oil in place of butter to roast and mash potatoes and sauté certain vegetables, because I like the flavour. Keep in mind, heating any oil changes and destroys its nutritional properties, especially if its smoking point has been reached. Coconut oil, though, does have many nutritional, antiviral, antibacterial, and antifungal properties when raw and unrefined.

While no cooking oil is a healthy oil, some oils are far better than others. I use raw coconut oil and olive oil both topically and in raw dishes and salad dressings. I cook with olive oil, macadamia oil, or avocado oil when I can find it. These oils are mostly monounsaturated fats, with very low saturated fat. The structure of the oils change once they reach their smoking point, but many people cook with olive oil, so it's about personal choice here. I prefer these oils because they use the whole kernel and fruit, rather than just the seed as seed oils do. I also do not like to consume vegetable oils, such as canola/rapeseed oil, sunflower oil, soybean oil, corn oil, rice bran oil, or cottonseed oil as they are high in omega-6s. These oils generally come from genetically-modified crops as well. Oils aren't a wholefood, so I always use small amounts. You can also substitute oil with water or vegetable broth to sauté or stir-fry.

Our bodies process wholefoods far better than part-foods and processed foods. It's important to get all of the essential nutrients from wholefoods.

The difference between brown rice and white rice is that brown rice contains seven layers of fiber on the outer surface, whereas, white rice has these layers stripped away. Because of this, brown rice is a wholefood that contains far more nutrients, but also contains more arsenic than white rice. Although arsenic is an essential ultra-trace mineral, it is suggested to eat brown rice only every now and then.

Fruit is full of essential vitamins, minerals, enzymes, and phytonutrients which are completely bioavailable and aren't found in other foods. Many people limit their fruit intake because of its sugar content, however, fruit, as a wholefood is digested differently than other sugars. Fiber is known to help control blood sugar levels. When fruit is eaten as a wholefood, the fiber helps slow down the absorption of carbohydrate sugars in the small intestine. This means that it helps prevent sharp spikes in blood sugar levels which aids in digestion, and excess sugars are then excreted from the body. However, if fruit doesn't agree with you, then there is more going on and fruit is merely a trigger, not the cause.

When properly fuelled, our bodies function at their peak, meaning that we shouldn't be scared of fruit. If the sugar content in fruit scares you or upsets your body somehow, then there is more going on. Insulin is regulated by many things and is part of the role that potassium and magnesium play in the body. Before writing off fruit, make sure that your gut health and micronutrient levels, which I will cover in the next chapter, are sufficient. Make sure you're eating organic produce, and finally, make sure that your saturated fat levels are lower.

Fruits are the foods that are the highest in lifeforce, ahead of vegetables and sprouted legumes and grains. This is because the majority of fruits grow on trees which receive large amounts of Sun, and 'Sun energy' is how lifeforce reaches us on Earth. Trees are also full of lifeforce, so when we eat their fruits, we not only eat a plethora of antioxidants, vitamins, minerals, and phytonutrients, but we are also consuming that Sun energy and lifeforce as well. While fruits and vegetables can maintain their Sun energy and lifeforce until they decompose, the fresher the fruit, the better!

This brings me to smoothies versus juicing. While I love to drink fresh cold-pressed juice from time to time, juice is still considered a part-food because a lot of the fruit is left behind, including the important fiber. Smoothies are a blended mix of whole fruits which means that our bodies absorb nutrients and digest smoothies far better than juice. In addition, our bodies digest the sugars differently after drinking juice versus a smoothie, and the sugars can cause distress to the pancreas. Opt for smoothies over juices, eat the skin when possible, and don't rely on fruit-based superfood powders for your fruit intake, as many of the nutrients, including the lifeforce, are lost during the processing stages.

With many superfood and fruit powders becoming more and more popular, make sure to check the country of origin first. Superfood powders including blue and green spirulina, pink pitaya powder, açaí powder, matcha, beetroot powder, baobab, maca, moringa, seabuckthorn, barley, and wheat grass, as well as fruit powders including mango, blueberry, strawberry, and wildberry, have flooded Chinese wholesale websites. It's all too easy for a brand to repackage these superfoods and resell them, and many of these brands don't list the country of origin on their websites. If in doubt, ask! It is crucial to know where sea vegetables and algae, well, all foods, are sourced from in case of contamination. Please also note that some sellers 'irradiate' their powders which means that they treat the food with radiation to make the colours brighter. Before coughing up ridiculous amounts of money for superfood powders check the country of origin and make sure the product is GMO-free, organic, and non-irradiated. True superfoods are whole fresh fruits and vegetables!

Frozen açaí also comes in different standards. Many brands blend the açaí seeds with the fruit pulp to fill the volume, however, the seeds are inedible! You may notice a brown-film on top of your smoothie, or you may not feel the best afterwards; you can thank the açaí seeds for that. Some of the largest açaí brands do this, as they purely focus on 'marketing' rather than the quality and integrity of their products.

This brings me to mock-meat. I love the concept of companies using plant-derived foods to make 'meat.' Every mock-meat patty, sausage and pie saves animals from being eaten, but from a wholefoods standpoint, mock-meats are a plethora of part-foods. And some even use toxic and GMO ingredients. There are a few cleaner brands around, but for the most part, they're more about flavour and texture than health. I personally prefer home-made patties and sausage rolls made from wholefoods, such as sweet potato, lentils, and beans.

When it comes to cruciferous vegetables like broccoli, cauliflower, Brussels sprouts, kale and cabbage, we can't actually digest these vegetables properly due to an indigestible sugar called *raffinose*. This is why cruciferous vegetables cause bloating and flatulence in many people. While I don't recommend cutting out these nutrient-dense foods, it is important to cook them properly to make them easier to digest. Steaming, quick blanching, stir-frying or pressure cooking are the recommended ways to cook these vegetables. And always opt for organic as these foods tend to be heavily sprayed. Although kale is a nutrient-powerhouse because it easily soaks up nutrients from the soil, it also means that it easily soaks up pesticides and herbicides too.

I am often asked about eating and encapsulating the placenta after birth because it supposedly contains a lot of nutrients. While this is true, the placenta also contains toxins. One of the placenta's functions is to act as 'baby's shield,' a line of defense if we become sick during pregnancy or encounter any toxins that we haven't been able to excrete. The placenta absorbs toxins, and colds and flus, so that they don't reach baby. Sadly, if there are too many toxins for the placenta to absorb, the toxins will penetrate and cross the placenta. You can ask any OB/GYN how they can tell if a mama has smoked during her pregnancy, without prior knowledge: the placenta has a smudgy-coating around the outside. High consumption of Coca-Cola during pregnancy is known to have the same effect too. Studies have also shown that smoker's placentas are heavier for the weight of their babies. With this in mind, don't eat the placenta. If you do not want your precious placenta to be thrown in the trash, take it home and bury it in the Earth and/or plant a tree. Many cultures do this, including my own.

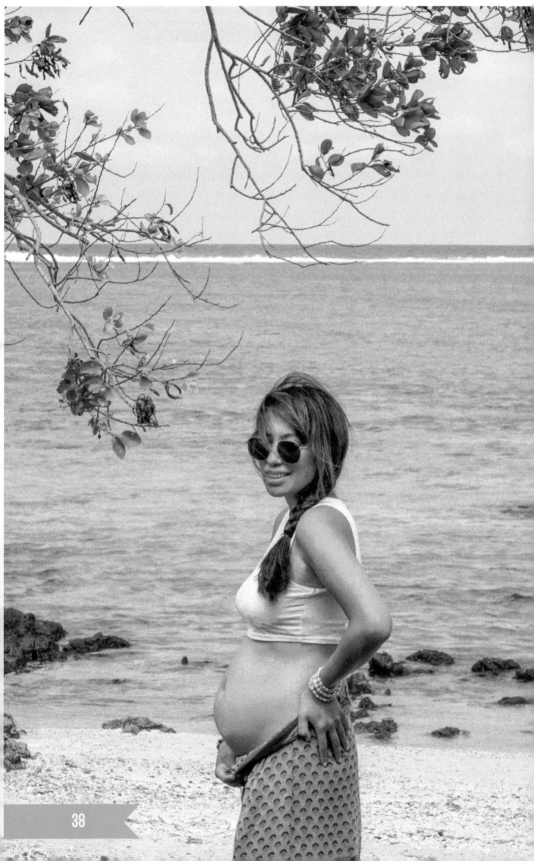

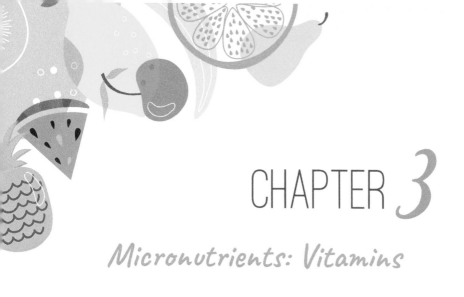

CHAPTER *3*

Micronutrients: Vitamins

Vitamins are organic nutrients — organic meaning there's a presence of carbon — that are essential in small doses for overall health and wellbeing. They are composed of carbon, hydrogen, oxygen, and sometimes nitrogen and cobalt. Each vitamin has a different arrangement of these elements and is considered essential if its removal from our diet compromises our health.

Most vitamins are obtained from the nutrients that we ingest, but some, including vitamin K2 (menaquinone) and some B vitamins, are produced by bacteria in the gut. Most of our vitamin D supply is made in our bodies when sunlight touches our skin and is also in some foods.

Fat-soluble vitamins include A, D, E, and K. These vitamins are usually stored in the liver or in the fat cells until needed. They are also better absorbed by the body if eaten with good fats.

Vitamin A (provitamin A) is converted in the body after eating the antioxidant, *beta carotene*, which is found in dark leafy vegetables, especially kale (contains almost 200% of the RDI) and other green, yellow, and orange foods such as apricots, carrots, pumpkin, mango, sweet potato, broccoli, watermelon, squash, and chlorella. Zinc, vitamin C, and vitamin E help enhance vitamin A absorption. *Retinol* is known as 'preformed Vitamin A,' because it is active and does not need to convert. This is only because it is found in animal products and has already been converted by the animal.

Vitamin D (a hormone) is produced in the body when we absorb sunlight, but we must be in the direct Sun and not behind a glass window. There is a lot of marketing about vitamin D supplements, but it is best produced in the body from exposure to the Sun. When we are exposed to sunlight, our bodies also produce and release the protein, GCMaF, which destroys cancer cells within the body and strengthens the immune system. We also absorb lifeforce from the Sun too. Vitamin D hormone supplements are a 'part-food' because of this.

During hotter months spend time in the Sun in the morning and before sundown, when the day is at its mildest temperatures. If you haven't spent much time in the Sun, build your time up slowly. Start with ten minutes, and then build up to fifteen minutes and go from there. When Kaimana was born, I started his exposure to the Sun when he was one-week-old, and I started with ten seconds. I made sure to expose the back of his body so his eyes were protected from the direct light. It's crucial to start off with brief exposure because baby has 'new skin' that hasn't been exposed to the Sun at all. As baby grows and begins to get used to the Sun, gradually increase his exposure.

Vitamin D stores in the body, so getting adequate Sun during the warmer months helps to get us through the cooler and wetter months. However, if Winter delivers sunny days, make sure to get at least ten minutes per day in the Sun!

There is such a thing as 'overexposure,' so make sure to be Sun smart. More on this in Chapter 7.

Mushrooms are also a great source of vitamin D, and if you leave mushrooms in the Sun, they will produce even more. This is because mushrooms are rich in the vitamin D precursor, *ergosterol*, which the Sun converts into vitamin D2. Vitamin D3 is made within the body when exposed to the Sun. There is no difference between these varieties in terms of raising blood levels of vitamin D, however, D3 is superior in sustaining those levels. Vitamin A, vitamin C, and calcium enhance vitamin D production and absorption.

Vitamin E is an antioxidant and is primarily found in oils, nuts, and seeds, and can be found in green leafy vegetables, avocados, mangoes, tomatoes, and sweet potatoes. Selenium, vitamin C, zinc, and copper enhance vitamin E absorption.

Vitamin K is known as the clotting vitamin because without it, our blood wouldn't clot. Vitamin K is also involved in the synthesis of bone proteins to ensure proper bone density. Vitamin K1 (phylloquinone) is found in foods like green leafy vegetables especially kale (contains about 10x the RDI) and collard greens, natto (fermented soy), Brussels sprouts, cabbage, broccoli, cucumbers, dried basil and oregano, kiwifruit, dates and prunes. Vitamin K2 (menaquinone) is found in fermented foods, it's produced by bacteria in the gut, and is also synthesized in the body from eating vitamin K1 foods.

Vitamin K2 also plays a role in protecting our teeth, and healthy intestinal bacteria which leads to good gut health, helping to enhance absorption. Menadione, also known as vitamin K3, is a synthetic version of vitamin K and is commonly used in pet food and supplements. It is also a vitamin K precursor, meaning that it is converted into vitamin K2 within the body. Early pregnancy nausea can be a sign of a vitamin K deficiency. Vitamin K doesn't always cross the placenta, and baby's vitamin K levels are dependent on your intake during pregnancy and while breastfeeding. During breastfeeding, our amazing mammary glands can also synthesize vitamin K, so make sure to keep up vitamin K-rich foods during pregnancy, especially in the final weeks, and while breastfeeding. A healthy baby will also begin to produce vitamin K within his gut after the first week of being born, and levels peak at around day seven or eight after birth.

In cases where baby may have issues producing vitamin K after the first week of birth could be due to several reasons, including preterm delivery, low birth weight, if mama used antibiotics, anticoagulants, anticonvulsants, and other medications during pregnancy, or undetected liver disease, amongst other reasons.

Menadione (vitamin K3) can interfere with the function of *glutathione*, one of the body's natural antioxidants, resulting in oxidative damage to cell membranes. Menadione given by injection has induced liver toxicity, jaundice, and hemolytic anemia in infants; therefore, menadione is no longer used for the treatment of vitamin K deficiency. Synthetic vitamin K1 (phytonadione) is now used instead.

Water-soluble vitamins are only stored in the body temporarily, with the exception of vitamin B12 and folate (B9), as these vitamins store in the liver. This group of vitamins include vitamin C and vitamin B-complex.

Vitamin C is found in citrus fruits, berries, kiwifruit, capsicum, tomatoes, broccoli, kale (contains 200% RDI) and sweet potatoes, among many other fruits and vegetables. As well as playing a crucial role in aiding our immune systems, vitamin C is an antioxidant, a natural antihistamine (some mild allergies are linked to vitamin C deficiency), and enhances the absorption of many other nutrients such as iron, vitamin A, vitamin D, vitamin C, and magnesium. Vitamin C also works with the B-vitamins to produce energy.

Vitamin B-complex is a group of vitamins including:

- **B1 (thiamin)** is found in nuts, mushrooms, oats, seeds, peas, sweetcorn, tomatoes, and oranges.

- **B2 (riboflavin)** is found in mushrooms, spinach, almonds, legumes, nuts, seeds, and quinoa.

- **B3 (niacin)** is found in mushrooms, potatoes, peanuts, and green vegetables such as peas, Brussels sprouts, asparagus, and bok choy.

- **B5 (pantothenic acid)** is found in mushrooms, legumes, avocado, broccoli, sweet potatoes, and some wholegrains.

- **B6 (pyridoxine)** is found in bananas, broccoli, mushrooms, potatoes, starchy vegetables, non-citrus fruits, legumes, nuts, and seeds.

- **B7 (biotin)**, also called vitamin H, is found in avocado, sweet potato, cauliflower, soy, legumes, mushrooms, and nuts.

- **B9 (folate)** is found in green leafy vegetables, mushrooms, beets, citrus fruits, Brussels sprouts, legumes, asparagus, broccoli, nuts, seeds, papaya, and chlorella. Please note that folic acid and folate are not the same. Folate is the natural vitamin, and folic acid is the synthetic version of folate. Folic acid has also been proven to be far less bioavailable than folate.

- **B12 (cobalamin)** is made by bacteria and is stored in the body, mainly in the liver. B12 is found in mushrooms, sea vegetables and seaweeds such as nori and chlorella. Some fermented foods contain B12 if the food producer has added the B12 bacteria to it, meaning that some kombuchas and sauerkrauts contain bioavailable B12.

Sea moss is a sea vegetable that's high in many nutrients including vitamins B2, B3, B5, B6 and B9. When sourcing sea vegetables, it is important to know where the food is sourced, due to pollution, such as the Fukushima radiation leak.

Vitamin B1, B6, and B9 deficiencies during pregnancy have been linked to toxaemia and stillbirths. While there are many reasons why stillbirths occur, these vitamin deficiencies have been linked to them.

What about supplements?

If you take a B12 supplement, please consider that the B-complex vitamins enhance the absorption of each other. This means that B6 helps the absorption of B12 and B9, and vice versa. If you're taking a B12 supplement without any of the other B vitamins, you are most likely not absorbing as much as you think. When it comes to supplements, most are concentrated part-foods or synthetic which are hard for our bodies to digest. My suggestion is to take a B-complex powder that is made from food.

Sea moss, sarsaparilla and chlorella are the main food powders that I keep in my house. I add sea moss to our smoothies, and I also make a nutritious hemp, sea moss and Medjool date milk as well! I also keep a food-made vitamin C powder handy in case of sickness or allergies. Other powders, such as barley grass, wheat grass, and spirulina are jam packed with micronutrients including some of the B-vitamins, potassium, zinc, iodine, iron, and vitamins A and C. These powders are an excellent addition to smoothies.

A lot of people ask me about nutritional yeast, and although nutritional yeast contains most of the B vitamins, I don't like how processed it is. Plus, most of the vitamins are added and synthetic as only B2/riboflavin is created during fermentation. This means that nutritional yeast is a poor source of bioavailable B vitamins. I also don't like to add yeast to any of my food. I will cover why in Chapter 10.

However, nature has provided us with a completely bioavailable B-complex food: mushrooms! In the 1980's and 1990's, mushrooms were labelled as 'the meat for vegetarians,' and it was common knowledge that they contained B12. However, as vegetarianism and veganism grew in popularity, all of a sudden, mushrooms contained no B12. Not too long ago, the University of Western Sydney studied mushrooms from five different mushroom farms around Australia and they all contained B12. The quantities of B12 varied between each farm, and the reported levels were low, so it isn't recommended to solely rely on mushrooms for B12. However, because mushrooms contain all of the B-vitamins, it makes these little fungi the perfect bioavailable B-complex food. Step outside of your comfort zone and try different varieties of mushrooms to eat a variety of nutrients. I have also gone into more detail about B12 producing in the gut in Chapter 5.

I do believe vegans aren't the only ones at risk of a B12 deficiency, as vegans are generally conscious of their B12 intake, whereas most non-vegans unthinkingly rely on meat, seafood, and eggs. B12 is mainly stored in the liver, not only in livestock but in us as well, meaning that the muscle part of the animal, which is usually what is eaten, isn't where most of the B12 is stored. Also, a large majority of the cows have little-to-no access to grass, meaning that they have little-to-no access to the B12 bacteria which lives in the soil under the grass. And, if the soil is already depleted, then it may not contain B12, or cobalt which is found inside B12. The same can be said for all animal meat and chicken's eggs. If the animal isn't eating the B12 bacteria, then eating that animal or its eggs aren't reliable sources of B12. It is said that some farmers inject B12 into the animals because of this.

Vitamin C is another supplement that many people take. It has become popular to take mega-doses of this vitamin to prevent colds and flus, and to heal illnesses. Here's the deal with vitamin C: because it is a water-soluble vitamin, it isn't stored in the body. Studies have shown that we only absorb up to around 200mg at a time. If you take a 1000mg tablet you are most likely only absorbing 200mg, and the rest is discarded in your urine. And chances are that the tablet is synthetic too. While I do love vitamin C, one orange provides 100% of our RDI but that doesn't mean to just eat one orange, and that's it. It is merely to highlight that we can easily eat enough vitamin C daily, whether pregnant or not. If you take a vitamin C supplement, if you have a mild allergy, or if you feel a cold or flu coming on, take two to three 200mg doses of a natural, food-made, vitamin C, spread out over the day, rather than one mega-dose of 1000mg.

While all vitamins and minerals are essential during pregnancy, the B-complex vitamins, vitamin C, vitamin D, vitamin E, and vitamin K are especially important. Increase vitamin-rich foods, spend time in the Sun, and use food-made supplements where necessary.

I am a huge fan of taking chlorella, spirulina, and/or barley grass during pregnancy, however, if you opt to take chlorella, try and start taking it before you become pregnant. Chlorella has powerful detoxing effects, and you want your body to be used to it before pregnancy. There has been concern about chlorella's detoxing effects and the redistribution of heavy metals from out of the bloodstream and/or fat cells, and possibly redistributing them to baby. Chlorella actually binds to the heavy metals in the intestines and gut, where they are then expelled in the faeces and urine. Chlorella can also help maintain iron levels during pregnancy and can help thicken the blood. This is particularly helpful if you have a history of losing a lot of blood during childbirth, or if your blood is thin. Chlorella has also been shown to reduce the levels of toxic dioxins in breast milk. I prefer to add half to one teaspoon of chlorella powder to coconut water, rather than adding it to smoothies because it overpowers them. Surprisingly, it doesn't taste too bad with coconut water. Please always check with your practitioner before starting any dosage.

With prenatal vitamins, many have been tested to show dangerous and unacceptable levels of toxic heavy metals including lead and aluminium. I do believe that we can gain plenty of essential nutrients through wholefoods, including sea moss, herbs and nutritional powders. However, if you need to take a prenatal vitamin, please research the brand and ingredients first, and opt for organic and food-made vitamins if possible.

Vitamin Inhibitors

This is the same with minerals, but the most common vitamin inhibitors are alcohol, coffee, caffeine, antibiotics, the contraceptive pill, fried foods, phytic acid, smoking, and refined sugars. When you're eating your main meals or nutrient-dense foods, try to avoid these common inhibitors directly before, during, and straight after meals.

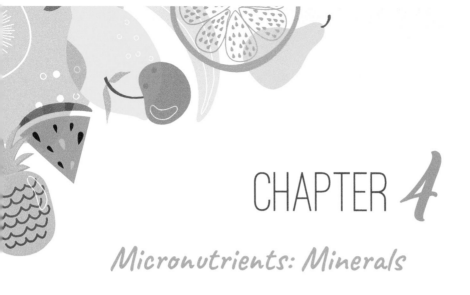

CHAPTER 4

Micronutrients: Minerals

Like vitamins, minerals are crucial to our wellbeing. Macro-minerals are essential minerals that our bodies need more of, and trace minerals are essential minerals that our bodies require in much smaller doses. Ultra-trace minerals are minerals that we require in the most minute doses and we generally get enough of them in a balanced diet.

MACRO-MINERALS

Calcium, Magnesium, Potassium, Phosphorus, Chloride, Sodium, and Sulfur.

TRACE MINERALS (micro-minerals)

Iron, Iodine, Manganese, Zinc, Chromium, Copper, Molybdenum, Cobalt, (Calcium) Fluoride, and Selenium.

ULTRA TRACE MINERALS

Nickel, Vanadium, Arsenic, Boron, and Silicon.

Calcium is the most abundant mineral in the body, with about 99% residing in our bones and teeth. Some calcium is in our blood, and our bodies will forfeit calcium from our bone and teeth stores if we aren't getting enough. This is why a blood test isn't always the best way to tell if someone has enough calcium in their body, as it only measures calcium in the blood. If you want to have your bone mineral measured properly, you can opt to have a DEXA (bone mineral density scan), but just be mindful that this is a full body x-ray and shouldn't be done during pregnancy.

Some of the best food sources for calcium are nuts, seeds (especially hemp and tahini), legumes, grains such as teff and amaranth, and leafy greens, home-made fortified milks, juices, cereals, and tofu. While I don't recommend using conventional cereals, juices, or milks as a trusted source of calcium, you can make your own milk and fortify it yourself. This way you know exactly how much has gone into it, and what the calcium source is, as calcium supplements can be made from oyster shell and bone meal. Typical fortified cereals and milks also use synthetic vitamins which are harder for the body to absorb, so opt for wholefood sources first. Another food source that is heavy in calcium, as well as iron, magnesium, and potassium, are sea vegetables, such as kelp noodles and sea moss. As previously mentioned, please be mindful of where the sea vegetables are sourced from.

Iron is yet another crucial mineral. Our bodies need iron to make red blood cells which transport oxygen through our bodies and is needed to maintain our energy levels. During pregnancy our bodies make up to 50% more blood, and baby also builds up his iron stores within his liver, which means that our need for iron increases. And because breast milk is made from mama's blood, iron is also crucial for breast milk production. Studies have shown that anaemic mama's have had insufficient milk supply.

If you have your full blood-count tested at the start of your pregnancy, your iron levels (haemaglobin) and iron stores (ferritin and haemosiderin) may be satisfactory. However, as you progress during pregnancy your body needs more iron. Have your iron tested near the end of your second trimester, when baby starts building his reserves, and again in your third trimester. An iron deficiency during pregnancy is common and can lead to complications during labour. If you experience dizziness, shortness of breath, constant fatigue, and/or Restless Leg Syndrome, please have your iron tested, as these are common symptoms of a deficiency/depletion.

If you happen to test low, eat more iron-rich foods and take an organic, bioavailable iron supplement until your iron levels improve. Iron fluorine is the iron found in plants, whereas, iron oxide – which is found in many supplements – comes from rocks and is harder for the body to absorb. An iron fluorine supplement typically comes in the form of dried herbs as a powder or a capsule. Opt for that if your practitioner deems it safe, and if it doesn't contain any herbs that you should avoid during pregnancy (try the Plantfed Mama Herb Shop). There is also new information about taking iron oxide tablets and their effect on the body, making it harder to absorb iron from food. Only take iron oxide supplements if absolutely necessary, when treating low levels or a deficiency.

You may need to continue taking the supplement until after you've finished bleeding or breastfeeding. Some iron oxide supplements cause constipation for mama (and baby if breastfeeding). If iron fluorine isn't a possibility for you, this can be avoided by taking an organic iron supplement that is combined with spinach and/or spirulina, making sure it is also combined with vitamin C. Herbs that help increase iron levels are sarsaparilla root, dandelion root, alfalfa (must be taken in smaller doses), and nettle, and all four can be taken as a tea and/or eaten while pregnant and breastfeeding. However, please check with your practitioner first.

There are two types of iron found in food: non-haem (iron that comes from plants), and haem iron (iron that comes from blood/animals). It has been said that non-haem iron is less bioavailable; however, recent studies have found links between haem iron, and diabetes and gestational diabetes. Researchers have also found that non-haem iron isn't associated with diabetes and that it is protective against diabetes. I have included the details of these studies further on.

Iron-rich plant-foods include nuts (especially pistachios), seeds (especially hemp seeds), and hemp protein powder, leafy greens, some grains, and legumes, such as black beans, kidney beans, soybeans, chickpeas, lentils, and peanuts, with soybeans, black beans, and kidney beans containing the most. Fortunately, there are ways to increase absorption by food pairing. Eating iron-rich foods with vitamin C-rich foods such as citrus fruits, berries, kiwifruit, capsicum, kale, tomatoes, and sweet potatoes will help increase iron absorption. I love how nature has given us iron-rich foods that we'd usually eat with vitamin C foods anyway. Legumes and salad, or hemp seeds/protein and fruit are the perfect combos! Chlorella, sea moss, and teff also contain iron and vitamin C.

Teff is a powerhouse gluten-free grain that is also high in iron — it contains more iron than meat — and contains vitamin C to naturally help absorption. I will go into more detail about increasing absorption and reducing mineral inhibitors in Chapter 8. However, if you are prone to iron deficiency, foods such as chocolate, soda, tea and coffee, and any foods that contain caffeine and high amounts of tannins, can deplete the body of iron. Caffeine has also been shown to decrease iron concentrations in breast milk, so please keep this in mind when breastfeeding.

One of the most important minerals that is often overlooked is magnesium. Magnesium is the fourth most abundant mineral in the body, behind calcium, phosphorus, and sulfur. Magnesium helps to maintain healthy teeth and bones, assists healthy nerve and muscle function, supports a robust immune system, and with the help of calcium, it helps to maintain a steady heartbeat. Magnesium also aids in the production of energy and protein, and assists in the removal of toxic waste from the body tissues.

Edema is common during pregnancy and it is associated with excess sodium in the body. Magnesium helps the removal of toxic waste from the tissues, and a magnesium deficiency can result in fluid build-up resulting in edema as well.

The cause of migraines can be because of too many heavy metals in the body, especially on the brain, but migraines are also associated with a magnesium deficiency as well.

Magnesium also helps regulate blood glucose levels, and together with potassium, both minerals assist in insulin secretion, which brings me to the link between magnesium and/or potassium deficiency and type-2 diabetes and gestational diabetes. Gestational diabetes can be caused by the hormonal changes in the body, but what we eat and what we don't eat, heavily affects our hormones.

While there are studies that have linked gestational diabetes to egg and bacon (haem-iron) consumption prior to pregnancy, and to saturated fat intake, there is also ongoing research into the role of magnesium in preventing and managing high blood pressure, heart disease, and even diabetes. Considering that two types of type-2 diabetes medications, *Pioglitazone* and *Metformin*, raise magnesium levels in the body, this supports the direct link between magnesium deficiencies and diabetes.

Studies have also shown that women with gestational diabetes who increased their magnesium intake showed improvement. While it takes more than magnesium to heal gestational diabetes, my recommendation is always prevention over cure, because what we eat, and what we don't eat, is a significant factor.

However, the current method to test for gestational diabetes is flawed. If mama doesn't eat refined sugars, then drinking the 'chemical sugar drink' which many contain bromate/brominated vegetable oil (and makes many mamas sick), can register as a false positive. This is because mama's body isn't used to synthetic chemicals and will react much differently after drinking the 'chemical sugar drink' than after eating her usual foods. Many mamas who have tested positive have reported that their blood sugar never spiked after eating their everyday foods. These mamas were also not overweight and did not have a history of diabetes in their families. Testing should commence after mama has eaten her usual foods, not after drinking a toxic chemical drink.

Other often overlooked trace minerals are manganese and molybdenum. These minerals can be found in leafy green vegetables, nuts, seeds, legumes, and wholegrains. Manganese is an essential element for bone formation and is necessary for growth, development, and normal functioning of our bodies. For example, a symptom of a manganese deficiency in children is growing pains. Manganese is also involved in the metabolism of carbohydrates, cholesterol, and amino acids. Molybdenum also works together with calcium, magnesium, and potassium to keep our bones and teeth healthy. A molybdenum deficiency is rare, but a deficiency will result in a uric acid build up, which brings about inflammation and sore and painful joints. The body requires only small amounts of both trace minerals and are best sourced through food.

Iodine is a trace mineral that is required by the body to make thyroid hormones and is especially important for those with hypothyroidism. The body needs thyroid hormones for proper brain and bone development during pregnancy and infancy. BVO (found in many gestational diabetes tests, soda/soft drinks, and is even used as a flame retardant) blocks the production of thyroid hormones. Food sources for iodine are sea vegetables (including the powerhouse nutrient-dense seaweed, sea moss), pink Himalayan salt, and cacao powder, and chocolate made from cacao. Artichokes, potatoes, spinach, watercress, turnips, peas, beans, corn, broccoli, and cauliflower contain iodine. Strawberries, cranberries, figs, pineapples, apples, coconuts, grapefruit, kiwis, rhubarb, mangoes, dates, prunes, and apricots also contain iodine.

Iodine levels depend on the iodine content in the soil, with higher levels in the soil and foods that grow close to the ocean. Like magnesium, iodine can also be absorbed through the skin, so if you live near the sea, go for regular swims.

Copper is also a forgotten yet important trace mineral. One of its many functions is that it works with iron to help make red blood cells! It also helps to maintain nerve cells and the immune system, it helps the body form collagen, and helps iron absorption as well. Food sources for copper are leafy greens, nuts and seeds, spirulina, sea vegetables, shiitake mushrooms and dark chocolate/cacao.

Selenium is an essential trace mineral that is also an antioxidant. It helps boost immunity and is essential for thyroid health, blood flow, and lowers the chance of heart disease. Food sources for selenium are Brazil nuts, beans, sunflower seeds, brown rice, shiitake mushrooms, lentils, bananas, and cashews. Only a small amount of selenium is required by the body and is best sourced through food. One Brazil nut can provide the RDI.

Harvard Nurses' Health Study found that eating meat before pregnancy appeared to increase subsequent diabetes risk during pregnancy, due to the carcinogenic nitrosamines in bacon which may be toxic to insulin-producing cells. An increased risk was also found in non-processed meat. Researchers then studied *glycotoxins*, the advanced glycation end products formed in meat, causing inflammation, which has been tied to gestational diabetes.

More recently, researchers studied animal-based, haem iron. Higher pre-pregnancy intake of dietary animal-based iron is associated with increased gestational diabetes risk. For type-2 diabetes, only animal-based iron was associated with diabetes risk. Plant-based iron, or non-haem iron, was not.

Researchers thought that this was because our bodies can't regulate the absorption of blood-based iron, and so, high intakes can lead to too much in the body. The same result was found for gestational diabetes. Blood-based or animal-based iron was associated with as much as triple the increased risk. However, plant-based haem-iron was found to be protective against diabetes. Which explains why pregnant women who eat vegan or vegetarian appear to be at a significantly lower risk of developing diabetes.

A recent Harvard study found that high pre-pregnancy consumption of animal fat and cholesterol were also associated with elevated gestational diabetes risk, which led researchers to believe that eggs increased the risk of diabetes during pregnancy. The more eggs women ate before getting pregnant and during early pregnancy, the higher their risk of developing diabetes during their pregnancies. These findings are consistent with other studies documenting associations with cholesterol intake and the development of type-2 diabetes in men and non-pregnant women. These studies can be found at www. nutritionfacts.org.

Another common complaint from pregnant women is cramps. Cramps are associated with a lack of electrolytes, such as potassium, magnesium, and/or sodium, but are more commonly potassium or magnesium. If you are suffering from cramps during pregnancy, try eating magnesium-rich foods and potassium-rich foods such as avocado, kiwifruit, bananas, apricots, oranges, coconut water, rockmelon (cantaloupe), grapefruit, potatoes, mushrooms, peas, cucumbers, zucchini, and even dates.

It is uncommon for people to suffer from sulfur and phosphorus deficiencies as many foods contain these minerals.

Another common outcome from pregnancy is stretch marks. Stretch marks occur because there is a lack of elasticity in the skin (and also because mama may be carrying a large baby or multiple babies). Zinc has an abundant role in our overall health, from helping our immune system, to healing wounds, to thyroid function, as well as aiding magnesium against diabetes, promoting muscle growth and repair, supporting liver health, and supporting skin elasticity, amongst many other functions. Zinc-rich foods are chickpeas, lentils, black beans, almonds, cashews, pepitas, spinach, and mushrooms.

Another tip to help skin elasticity is collagen, and collagen is plentiful in a wholefoods diet. High vitamin C fruits have the ability to help the amino acids, *lysine* and *proline*, convert collagen. Orange fruits and vegetables such as oranges, sweet potatoes and carrots, and kale, are loaded with vitamin A which also restores damaged collagen.

Added fluoride (in tap water and toothpaste) should be avoided as it is either *sodium fluoride* or *silicofluorides*. These fluorides are made up of toxic waste by-products from the phosphate fertilizer and aluminium industries. Natural fluoride is *calcium fluoride*, and this fluoride naturally occurs in soil and spring water.

Calcium is the antidote to fluoride poisoning, and when bound to fluoride in water, the calcium binds to and removes the fluoride from the body before it stores and causes harm. However, with sodium fluoride and silicofluorides, they completely fall apart in water, leaving the fluoride to store in the body. This topic is controversial because we have been told that fluoride is essential for our teeth, but the information that has been left out is that it isn't calcium fluoride that is added to the tap water. As you have previously read, many other vitamins and minerals play a crucial role in the health of our teeth. I will go into more detail in Chapter 16.

What about supplements?

I'm a huge believer that many ailments and illnesses begin due to a lack of minerals, vitamins, and nutrients in the body. Thus they can be reversed and even prevented, however, most supplements are concentrated part-foods or synthetic, and are tough for the body to digest and absorb. So, we shouldn't rely solely on supplements.

Many people assume that they can continue eating empty calories because they take a multi-vitamin, but supplements do not always work. Only some supplements are made from wholefoods, but mostly, they are made in a laboratory from synthetic ingredients, unethical ingredients, or ingredients with low bioavailability. Our bodies do not absorb concentrated, synthetic ingredients the same way as wholefoods. Which is why supplements made from wholefoods are much safer and far more effective. Wholefoods are balanced, and are easier to digest and absorb, which also increases bioavailability. If bioavailability of any supplement is low, then nutrients aren't adequately absorbed, thus being wasteful, which I call, 'wasteful supplementing.'

Remember that minerals do store in the body and unless there is a deficiency which requires 'essential supplementing,' daily concentrated mineral supplements are unnecessary and can be dangerous. While nutritional deficiencies are the beginning of many illnesses, it's important to utilize supplements correctly. If you need to add more nutrients to your diet and are finding it difficult through diet alone, opt for supplements made from wholefoods, while also eating an array of wholefoods.

Most supplements are made by extracting the mineral away from the food, and is then added to the supplement in concentrated doses. This is the term that is coined 'concentrated part-food.' However, many supplements aren't made from food at all, as many are extracted from inedible matter, such as rocks and coral reefs. Taking large and concentrated doses of mineral supplements, like calcium for example, can lead to hypercalcemia, a condition that weakens the bones. It also leads to too much calcium in the blood and can create kidney stones.

Taking concentrated supplements can also lead to a 'secondary deficiency'. This happens when there is too much of one mineral in the body, and it impairs the absorption of another mineral. For example, large doses of iron restrict zinc absorption. Large doses of calcium impair magnesium absorption. Too much zinc limits copper absorption. Too much calcium and phosphorus can limit manganese absorption, and iron and magnesium can limit phosphorus absorption. This is nature's way of protecting us from eating too many minerals, essentially, to protect us from overdosing. When we take large doses of a concentrated mineral, it creates an imbalance of the other minerals in the body. It's always best to gain nutrients through wholefoods, and, if a supplement is required, take a supplement made from wholefoods.

Make sure to increase calcium-rich foods like beans, lentils, leafy greens, hemp seeds, flax seeds, almonds, tofu/tempeh, amaranth, teff, and sea vegetables. If you have tested low in calcium, or if you know that you're not getting enough calcium in your diet, supplement with a powder that is made from food like sea vegetables, which has higher bioavailability. Instead of taking one large dose, spread the dosage out over two or even three applications, and fortify your own foods.

Add calcium powder or sea moss to your milk and fortify it yourself. The body needs to adjust to taking supplements and taking a mega-dose puts extra strain on the organs, and it will not be adequately absorbed.

If you experience heartburn during pregnancy, home-made calcium-fortified plant-milk will help ease the burn. Keep in mind what food triggered the heartburn and limit that food. Common triggers are often acidic foods including some grains, cooked tomato and spicy foods, greasy foods, carbonated drinks, and lying down too soon after eating.

Sea vegetables are a powerhouse food. Sea moss in particular, boasts incredible healing properties and nutrients, such as calcium, magnesium, iron, potassium, phosphorus, zinc and iodine, as well as vitamins A, B-complex (including folate), C, D, E and K. It's also a great source of Omega-3! Sea moss has unjustly received a bad reputation amongst some people in the health industry because it contains *carrageenan*, however, what most do not consider is that carrageenan (often used as a thickener and stabilizer in health foods) is a part-food – sea moss is a wholefood. Also, when you dig around and take a look at the studies that discredit carrageenan, there is only one researcher that discredits it, yet, study after study has found it to be safe. As previously mentioned, just be mindful of where your sea vegetables come from as some countries are not testing sea vegetables that may have been affected by the Fukushima radiation leak. Fake sea moss has also entered the market. Always look for purple sea moss powder, preferably from Canada, rather than white raw sea moss, as it's the raw sea moss that's been replaced by 'plastic sea moss' in many cases.

Diets high in protein and calcium increase the need for magnesium, so it is important not to take too much of any nutrient.

I do not recommend taking oral (concentrated) magnesium supplements as magnesium is best absorbed through the skin. Regardless if you have tested low in magnesium or not, increase magnesium-rich foods like spinach, quinoa, almonds, cashews, black beans, peanuts, hemp seeds, edamame/tofu/tempeh, and if possible, swim in the ocean regularly. The sea is an abundant and natural source of magnesium that is easily absorbed through the skin. That is why it is rare to hear of regular surfers and ocean swimmers with type-2 diabetes. Soaking in the ocean for at least thirty minutes can also help alleviate aches and pains. Every time I had lower back pains or typical pregnancy aches, I went for a casual ocean swim, and I swear by this method.

If swimming in the ocean isn't a possibility for you, add magnesium flakes — opt for magnesium chloride over magnesium sulfate — to a warm bath and treat yourself to a nice long soak. Alternatively, if you are low in magnesium, you can purchase a magnesium chloride spray from your local health shop and apply it to the skin as required. Many iron-rich herbs also contain high levels of magnesium as well.

While all vitamins and minerals are essential during pregnancy, calcium, magnesium, iron, zinc, and iodine are especially important. Be mindful of increasing these mineral-rich foods and use food-made supplements where necessary.

I hope this gives you a clear understanding of how we can easily incorporate adequate minerals into our diet, and the difference between 'essential supplementing' and 'wasteful supplementing.' Eat a wide range of fresh fruits, fresh vegetables, sea vegetables, safe herbs, soaked or activated nuts, legumes and seeds, and some wholegrains, and you'll eat the essential minerals that you need. And remember, stay clear of the substances that inhibit absorption before, during, and straight after meal times.

I've included the pregnancy and lactation RDIs (Recommended Daily Intake) for vitamins, minerals and some macronutrients on the following page, but I personally don't follow them. Minerals, B12, folate, and fat-soluble vitamins store in the body, so RDIs can be misleading. RDIs can also vary from country to country, and person to person, plus many RDIs are estimated due to limited research. Please only use these numbers as a guide. There are some nutrient calculators online where you can insert your age, and whether you're pregnant or not, and the calculator will give you an RDI estimate. Always talk to your health practitioner if you have any concerns.

MINERALS	RDI	VITAMINS	RDI
Magnesium	300-360mg	Vitamin B1	1.2-1.4mg
Potassium	2800mg 3200mg (lactation)	Vitamin B2	1.2-1.4mg 1.3-1.6mg (lactation)
Iron	23-27mg	Vitamin B3	14-18mg 13-17mg (lactation)
Calcium	900 - 1300mg	Vitamin B5	5mg 6mg (lactation)
Iodine	160-220mcg 270mcg (lactation)	Vitamin B6	1.6-2mg
Zinc	8.5-11mg 12mg (lactation)	Vitamin B7	30mcg 35mcg (lactation)
Selenium	55-65mcg 75mcg (lactation)	Vitamin B9	520-600mcg 450-500mcg (lactation)
Manganese	5mg	Vitamin B12	2.2-2.6mcg 2.8mcg (lactation)
Molybdenum	40-50mcg	Vitamin K	60mcg
Sodium	460-920mg	Vitamin C	40-60mg 80mg (lactation)
Protein	47 - 60g 51 - 67g (lactation)	Vitamin D	5mcg
Lipids	10g Linoleic acid + 1g ALA 12g Linoleic acid + 1.2g ALA (lactation)	Vitamin A	550-800mcg 1100mcg (lactation)

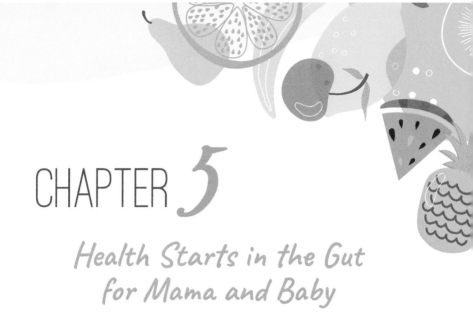

CHAPTER 5

Health Starts in the Gut for Mama and Baby

In recent years, more and more studies are showing the importance of gut health, and we now better understand just how crucial it is. Studies have also shown that how baby is born, and what baby is fed during infancy, also determines baby's microbiome, or gut health.

About 70% to 80% of our immune system resides in the digestive tract. The gut is where bacteria and the immune system meet. Effectively, much of our immunity resides in our gut, and experts have called it 'our second brain.' Although serotonin, the 'happy chemical,' is a brain neurotransmitter, approximately 90% of the body's serotonin is made in the digestive tract. Thus, there is a direct link between gut health and mental health.

With this in mind, we don't pay enough attention to baby's gut health. Baby's gut health is baby's immunity defense. In other words, if baby has a strong gut, then baby will also have a strong immune system. Breast milk naturally contains probiotics, but if you have to formula feed, speak to your holistic practitioner about administering probiotics as well. A powder form will be easy to mix into the formula or into baby's bottle. Also, be mindful of what oral medications baby takes as well, as these can compromise baby's gut.

A compromised gut comes from an imbalance in gut flora. Probiotics are good bacteria that line the digestive tract and support our bodies ability to absorb nutrients and fight infection. Because a compromised gut loses the ability to absorb nutrients, most illnesses stem from poor gut health and poor digestion. This in turn means that we digest and expel our food far too slowly, leaving it to sit in the gut to rot and decay. This is also the link between our bodies being able to expel toxins or hold on to toxins. Our stomachs, small intestines and large intestines decide whether to absorb a substance or send it down to the colon for excretion. If our digestive tract is compromised, then we may absorb and store toxins, rather than get rid of them.

In a compromised gut, toxins can be absorbed into the bloodstream, before being deposited all over the body, in our fat cells, our mouths/gums, and in our organs including our brains. Conversely, it compromises our ability to absorb the nutrients that we need. If we're holding on to toxins, our lymphatic system and liver are constantly working overtime, and we can hold on to toxins for years. These stored toxins then manifest as cancerous growths and tumours, amongst many other ailments.

Our bodies are so incredibly smart and will do almost anything to keep these toxins from causing harm by either expelling the toxins through excretion or vomiting. If the gut is compromised, then the body has trouble expelling toxins, so it does the next best thing: it stores the toxins in our fats cells which is where they will cause the least amount of harm. If we're underweight or if our fat cells contain a lot of toxins or other various reasons, then our bodies can begin to store the toxins all around the body, including our organs.

When the digestive tract is functioning poorly, our bodies not only have trouble eliminating toxins, but the immune system becomes compromised as well. This is where illness and disease come in.

While our bodies have the amazing ability to heal, if the gut is compromised and we don't make any modifications, then nothing will change. So, what compromises our gut health?

Antibiotics. While these medications kill particular pathogens, antibiotics also kill good gut bacteria as well. Antibiotics do play a vital role in many instances; however, it is important to take antibiotics only when absolutely needed and take probiotics when on a course of medication.

Alcohol. This highly acidic liquid puts stress on the liver and the entire digestive system. While you've hopefully given up alcohol throughout your pregnancy, it is recommended to limit your intake after pregnancy, especially when breastfeeding too.

Candida Overgrowth. Beneficial bacteria in the digestive tract helps to keep candida from overgrowing, but in an already compromised gut, this yeast can overgrow and destroy gut health. While it isn't recommended to start a detox program during pregnancy, eliminating foods that feed this yeast is crucial: refined sugar, refined carbohydrates, yeast-containing foods, trans-fats, long-life products, and foods that are susceptible to mould. Eating raw coconut oil, papaya, and probiotic-rich (yeast-free) foods will also help.

Coffee/Caffeine. Another highly acidic liquid that puts stress on the body. Known as a diuretic, many say that coffee has a tonne of health benefits. However, being a diuretic, coffee should be looked at as 'medicinal' rather than consumed daily. Diuretics are diuretics because once taken, the body does whatever it can to expel it, and whatever is in the gut, from the body. You've probably given up coffee during your pregnancy, but this is something to keep in mind afterwards. Personally, I love the smell and taste of coffee, but I dislike what it does to my body. It makes me feel hungover after drinking it, and it took me a long time to give it up because coffee tastes soooo good! Please also remember that caffeine is a nutrient inhibitor in mama, and also decreases iron concentrations in breast milk.

Gluten. While some people can tolerate gluten a lot better than others, gluten is inflammatory and is hard on the digestion. Especially gluten from GMO grains. Too much gluten can lead to an imbalance in good gut bacteria, especially if it is pesticide-sprayed and non-organic.

Over-sanitation. Antibacterial sprays and gels kill all of the bacteria, both the bad and the good.

Parasites. Most people have parasites in their digestive tract, and while it can go mostly unnoticed, parasites are a cause of and reason for poor gut health. Like candida, it isn't recommended to start a detox program while pregnant, but limit foods that parasites thrive on: refined sugar, refined carbohydrates, processed foods, and gluten. Eating raw coconut oil, papaya, pineapple, raw garlic (if it isn't a food aversion for you), and probiotic-rich foods will help as well.

Processed foods and refined sugars. These are amongst some of the hardest foods for our bodies to digest. Foods that are hard to digest put unnecessary stress on the digestive system and kidneys. Eaten every now and then the body can cope, but if consumed regularly, the gut becomes compromised.

Painkillers. Non-steroidal anti-inflammatories have been known to inflame the gut lining. Gut inflammation compromises the digestive tract. If you need an anti-inflammatory, try adding ginger to your morning smoothie, drinking fresh ginger tea, or adding turmeric to your stir-fry.

Pesticides and herbicides (and glyphosate). Many GMO and non-organic foods have been found to destroy the healthy bacteria within the gut. Always eat organic or uncertified organic, spray-free, where possible, and don't be afraid to buy watermelon or oranges with seeds in them.

Stress. When we are stressed, our bodies release the body's primary stress hormone, *cortisol*. Too much cortisol in the body is detrimental to physical health, including gut health, as it negatively influences the microbiome causing gut inflammation. This stress response can also weaken the gut lining, resulting in illness, exhaustion and nutritional deficiencies. The inflammation inhibits the absorption of nutrients which can result in compromised immunity. If you are feeling stressed, take some 'me time.' Spend some time in nature, in the Sun, in the ocean, and don't be afraid to take naps! Naps are so important during pregnancy because sleeping helps our bodies heal and restore. Also, remember to breathe deeply; I will cover the importance of breathing properly in Chapter 12.

Water. Unfiltered, chlorinated, and fluoridated water can destroy beneficial gut bacteria, which creates an imbalance. Filter your water, drink natural spring water, and add a filter to your showerhead.

Gastro. This one absolutely sucks, especially during pregnancy. Our immunity is much lower during pregnancy, so it is much easier to catch illnesses like gastro. If you do happen to catch it, like I did in my fifth week, it is a long healing process, but it does heal! Drinking water probably won't be your most favourite thing to do, so even if you can't eat or drink water, drink coconut water. It is much more palatable when you're sick and it's full of necessary electrolytes. These electrolytes are crucial, and it'll fuel you, and baby, with essential nutrients while your system is compromised. And rest, rest, rest!

Once the gastro symptoms go, the gut is incredibly compromised, so eating can be difficult, but it's manageable. Eat plainer foods and stay away from foods that are hard to digest such as gluten, and cruciferous vegetables like cauliflower and broccoli, cold/frozen foods and processed foods, and take a pre/probiotic every day. Be mindful of using a metal teaspoon to mix the probiotic into food, as the metal can disrupt activated probiotics. It's important to be patient. Gastro is such a shock to the system and it will take a few weeks to fully recuperate. When you're on the mend, slowly add the cruciferous and frozen foods back to your diet when you're ready. If you experience a dull pain in your stomach not long after eating, reassess what you've eaten, and eliminate that food for the time being, and reintroduce that food later on. It will help to keep a food diary as well.

After recovering from sicknesses such as the flu or gastro, our bodies may take a little while to get back to normal, but on the bright side, we come out cleaner and clearer as well. Our pregnant bodies will try and get rid of any muck that shouldn't be there, and this may result in similar symptoms as a cold or flu. If you happen to fall sick, take note of how you feel once you recover.

For years, I have believed that we can gain every essential nutrient from plants and from the Sun without having to supplement them. But what I lacked was proof, particularly when it came to B12. I couldn't believe that we 'needed' animals or supplements to gain this crucial nutrient. Further studies are required, however, B12 bacteria has been shown to be synthesized by small intestinal bacteria, which means we not only produce the bacteria but we can absorb it as well. This comes after researchers believing that B12 was only synthesized by bacteria in the colon, which was why humans were theorized not to be able to absorb it. Having a healthy gut does show a promising role in bioavailable B12 naturally producing in the gut. Our bodies very much rely on our gut being healthy!

Probiotics have been within our systems since birth, and how we are born and what we are fed as infants determines our gut microbiome.

We have always been told that, at birth, baby's entire intestinal tract is completely sterile, and studies have shown that baby's gut is first colonized by maternal and environmental bacteria during birth and continues to be populated through feeding and other contacts. However, in recent studies scientists have been able to detect bacteria in the amniotic fluid, in the placenta, and in the fetus' intestines, supporting the idea that baby's microbiome starts in utero. It's possible that bacteria from mama's mouth travels through the bloodstream to reach the developing baby through the placenta. Or microbes may travel up from mama's vagina and into the womb. This means that mama's health – and the microbes that she may harbour – matter more for baby's microbiome development than scientists once thought.

Maternal diet, delivery method and feeding method influences baby's gut microbiome.

It isn't as simple as saying vaginal birthed, breastfed babies have more microbiome, but there is a vast difference between the types of bacteria between these babies.

One particular study reviewed 102 newborns: seventy babies were delivered via vaginal birth, and thirty-two babies were delivered via caesarean. In the first six weeks, seventy babies were exclusively breastfed, twenty-six babies received a combination of formula and breast milk, and six babies were exclusively formula fed. At the end of the six-week period, there was a significant difference in microbiome between delivery mode and feeding mode. Babies who were combination fed, that is both breast milk and formula, showed similar microbiome as babies who were exclusively formula fed.

Microbiome Genus	Overall (n=102) (%)	Vaginally delivered (n=70) (%)	Delivered by C-section (n=32) (%)	Exclusively breastfed (n=70) (%)	Combination fed (n=26) (%)	Exclusively formula fed (n=6) (%)
Bacteroides	26.4	34.6	20.7	27.9	22.1	28.8
Bifidobacterium	22.5	23.3	17.4	25.5	16.8	11.4
Streptococcus	13.8	12.1	14	11.7	18.7	16.9
Clostridium	7.9	5.1	8.8	6.8	11.9	2.4
Enterococcus	5.7	4.3	8.7	4.8	6.1	14.6
Blautia	3.6	2.7	5.5	1.8	7.1	9.4
Veillonella	3.4	3.6	4.6	3.5	3.2	2.9
Lactobacillus	3	2.5	4.2	3.4	2.8	0
Staphylococcus	2.6	1.6	3.4	3.3	1.2	0.1
Planococcus	2	1.4	2.9	1.5	3.3	2.6
Other genera	9.1	8.8	9.8	9.8	6.8	10.9

(Courtesy of US National Library of Medicine National Institutes of Health)

"Caesarean delivery has been associated with an increased risk of obesity, asthma, celiac disease and type-one diabetes, whereas breastfeeding has been related to decreased risks of asthma, obesity, infection, metabolic syndrome, and diabetes, among other illnesses, compared with formula feeding. While the mechanics for this aren't well understood, there is growing evidence linking exposure to microflora that is present during vaginal delivery, with the microbiome in infants. Moreover, following delivery, breast milk primes and matures the infant gastrointestinal system, and is believed to promote a unique microbial colonization profile. The specific microbes may be permanently affected by exposure to maternal vaginal microflora and/or to breast milk, and could represent a key mechanism to the underlying differences in immune development." *(Courtesy of US National Library of Medicine National Institutes of Health)*

Another study showed that what mama eats impacts baby's microbiome as well. It showed that maternal fruit intake was associated with infant gut microbial-community structure, and maternal dairy intake was associated with a different strain.

By the end of the first year of life, the microbial profile is distinct for each infant. By the age of 2.5 years, the microbiota fully resembles the microbiota of an adult in terms of composition.

While it is always mama's decision on how to deliver baby, and whether to breastfeed or formula feed, it is important to note these studies because it comes back to gut health. Not only are we responsible for our own gut health, but our decisions during pregnancy and infancy affect baby's gut health too.

Probiotics, especially the *Lactobacillus* strains, enhance the integrity of the intestinal barrier, which may result in maintenance of immune tolerance. Because of our lower immunity during pregnancy it is recommended to take a probiotic. I prefer to take shelf-stable probiotics because probiotics that must be kept in the fridge are more prone to destabilizing when heated in the digestive tract.

Members of the genus *Lactobacillus*, which is part of the order *Lactobacillales*, also help break down milk proteins present in breast milk and aids baby's digestion. Recent evidence has shown that *Lactobacillus reuteri,* a probiotic that can be found in breast milk and in the gut microbiome, can help alleviate symptoms of colic. Or more so, the lack of *Lactobacillus reuteri* in baby's gut can result in colic. It is also *Lactobacillus reuteri* that is one of the bacteria that has been shown to help produce B12 in the gut.

For mamas who used antibiotics prior to delivery, the normal oral microbiome of the developing baby is disturbed by the expansion of *Proteobacteria*, which decreases the numbers of *Lactobacillales*. This means that the use of antibiotics produces bacteria that kills the good probiotic bacteria that baby needs to break down milk proteins. This results in poor digestion which can lead to gastrointestinal issues and colic.

Bifidobacterium lactis is another 'good bacteria' strain that's found in healthy newborns and breastfed infants. It's typically found in the gastrointestinal tract and in women's vaginas, which is why vaginal-birthed babies have higher amounts in their gut. *Bifidobacterium* were also reduced after the use of antibiotics and were replaced by the expansion of *Enterobacteriaceae,* which has the potential to become pathogenic under certain environmental conditions. *Enterobacteriaceae* are typically not regarded as probiotics. This means that mama's antibiotic use prior to birth destroys crucial probiotics that baby needs.

As you can see from the previous chart, breastfed babies had more than twice the amount of *Bifidobacterium* bacteria than formula fed babies. Exclusively formula fed babies also had zero *Lactobacillus* bacteria.

Prebiotics, a type of non-digestible fiber from plants, and resistant starches are what these probiotics feed on throughout the digestive tract. Our bodies can't break down prebiotics or resistant starches, so these foods can make their way through the digestive system, feeding the probiotics along the way.

Whether you have gut issues or not, it's still important to be mindful of your probiotic and prebiotic intake. However, I do believe that it is important to allow your body to make these beneficial bacteria without solely relying on a probiotic supplement. Take a probiotic until you feel confident that your gut-health is strengthening. It is also important to eat a variety of different plants as it's this variety that encourages healthy bacteria growth in the gut. And if you can, add probiotic foods to most meals. Fermented foods such as sauerkraut, fermented vegetables, and coconut yogurt are just three examples of probiotics in foods. Raw asparagus, unripe (green) bananas, and raw Spanish onion are just a few examples of prebiotics. Green bananas, oats, legumes, and cooked potatoes and rice that have been cooled down, are examples of resistant starch.

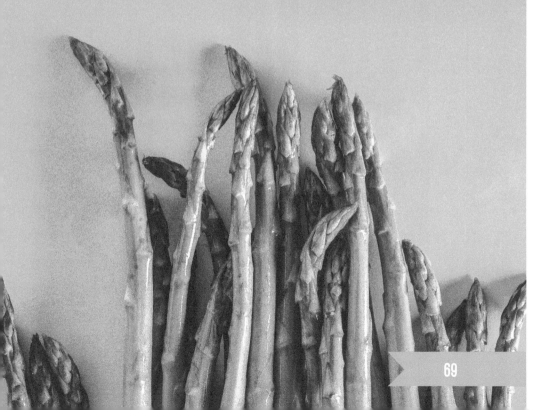

Want baby to eat vegetables later? Then eat yours now! Research has shown that babies who were exposed to certain tastes in utero were more eager to eat foods with the same tastes after birth!

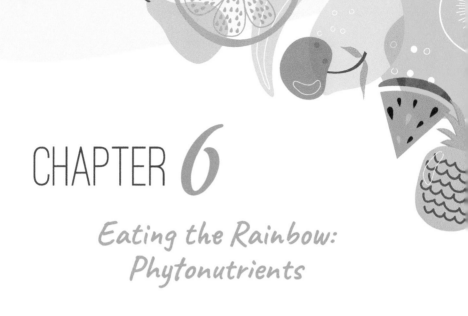

CHAPTER 6

Eating the Rainbow: Phytonutrients

Phytonutrients are nutrients that are derived from plants and are essential to life. They have the capacity to protect the human body and our cells from disease, pollutants, and UV radiation. In nature, phytonutrients are designed to promote the health and wellbeing of plants. Modern science is only just beginning to understand the crucial role that phytonutrients play in human health.

There are three ways that phytonutrients can assist human health:

- by changing the behaviour of free radicals
- by interacting with enzymes
- by adding hormones

One of the most widely researched phytonutrients are the antioxidants. Oxidation (oxidants) is the loss of an electron and occurs due to free radicals, reactive oxygen species (ROS), and oxidative stress. Inflammation caused by injury, over-exposure to UV light, radiation, smoking, and air pollution are all sources of free radicals. Free radicals can be generated both within the body and outside of the body, meaning in our environment.

Essentially, free radicals are searching for an electron, and issues arise if the free radical oxidizes LDL (bad cholesterol), proteins, or DNA in our bodies.

What these incredible antioxidants do, is that they 'give one for the team.' They give a donation of an electron from the antioxidant to a free radical in order to regenerate a stable compound, converting them back to harmless oxygen. Donating an electron is how vitamins and phytonutrients act as antioxidants. Minerals are co-factors for antioxidant enzymes.

While hundreds of phytonutrients are yet to be discovered, phytonutrients in broccoli and similar vegetables also act on specific enzymes within the body. They bind with, and remove, Phase-1 enzymes within the body, which can interact with cancer-causing toxins that naturally accumulate in the body and are thought to reduce a person's risk of developing cancer.

Phytonutrients are also recognized to interact with the human hormones. Dehydroepiandrosterone (DHEA) is one of the most important human hormones because it can convert itself to one of the other varieties of essential hormones including estrogen, progesterone, testosterone, and corticosterone, as required by the body. And as you might imagine, a deficiency in this hormone (which is common in the western world) causes hormonal imbalances which can wreak havoc on our health. DHEA is made from good cholesterol (HDL), and our body makes HDL from good fats. Eating nuts, avocados, raw coconut oil, olive oil, and hemp seeds will promote DHEA production within the body.

Look at the vast selection of fruits and vegetables and the beautiful colours that they show-off. Within these different plant foods and colours are different groups of phytonutrients, each with its vital role to keep us healthy! If we are eating the rainbow, eating a wide selection and colours from various plants, we are not only eating wholefoods, but we are also eating as many essential phytonutrients as we can.

!!EAT THE RAINBOW!!

FRUIT IS THE TRUE SUPERFOOD

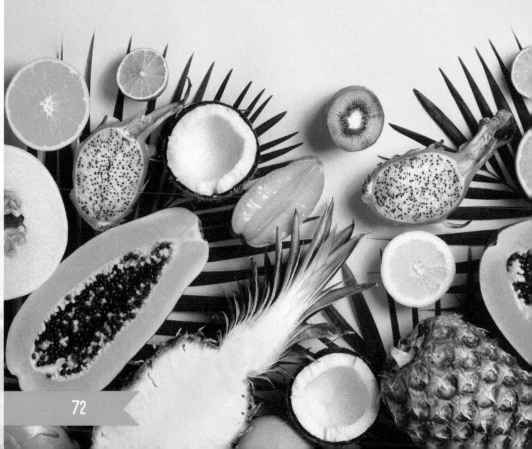

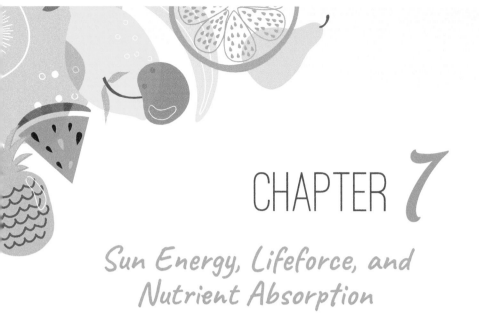

CHAPTER 7

Sun Energy, Lifeforce, and Nutrient Absorption

The Sun is one of my absolute favourite beings. The Sun gives us life, warmth, solar energy, and vitamin D. Vitamin D enhances our nutrient absorption, especially calcium and magnesium.

When our bodies produce vitamin D from the Sun, our bodies release a protein called GCMaF. This protein has been said to help the immune system destroy cancer cells and illnesses within the body. Credible studies have reported that GCMaF does show a promising role in cancer immunotherapy. That is why it is crucial to obtain vitamin D from the Sun and not to rely on supplements. You could say that this method is a 'wholefood' because you also produce GCMaF, while producing vitamin D, the way nature intended. Supplements are solely the concentrated hormone, vitamin D, minus GCMaF production.

Energetically and spiritually, lifeforce streams down to us on Earth via the Sun. The Sun is the reason why life and lifeforce exist here. When the Sun's energy, 'Sun energy', shines on animals, trees and plants, it transfers that Sun energy and lifeforce into them. That is the same for us!

Lifeforce, also called 'chi' and 'prana,' has been spoken of for thousands upon thousands of years. Like every living being we need lifeforce to survive. Without lifeforce we wouldn't be alive. The more lifeforce we have, the healthier and higher vibrational we are. If we are low on lifeforce then we will be sick, tired, and low vibrational.

We can absorb lifeforce directly from the Sun but we should be in the direct Sun and not behind a glass window. The Sun energy needs to touch our skin directly. In warmer months or when the Sun is at its hottest, spend time outside in the morning and in the evening. And always be sun-smart as there is such a thing as 'overexposure.'

If you're out in the Sun during the day wear a hat rather than sunglasses. Blocking the eyes with sunglasses tells the brain that we're indoors, and this message relays to our skin, making it easier to get burnt. If we keep our eyes uncovered, then the brain knows we're outside, and this message relays to our skin, meaning that our skin is prepared to be in the Sun. Try to use a hat only on baby as well.

And yes, sunscreen does block Sun energy from touching our skin. My family and I use coconut oil and olive oil as sunscreen, but we're also sun-smart. In summertime (when Sydney is super-hot and burny) we put 'clean' sunscreen on our faces and/or shoulders if we plan on being in the Sun for a while, and we always wear hats and rash vests. We also make sure that we get plenty of Sun all year round, so if we cover up on certain days, it doesn't matter too much.

While nutrients are a key to health and wellbeing, lifeforce is the major key. We've covered vitamins, minerals, wholefoods and phytonutrients and how to eat them, however, lifeforce foods are how we gain more lifeforce.

The foods highest in lifeforce are fruits, especially fruit that has grown on trees, and not far behind fruit, are vegetables, and sprouted legumes and sprouted wholegrains. Fruits contain the most lifeforce because fruit grows on trees, and trees have spent years in the Sun absorbing their own lifeforce, as well as absorbing lifeforce from the Earth. When trees grow their beautiful fruits, their fruits also spend a lot of time in the Sun.

Once I realized how much lifeforce was in raw and sprouted foods, especially fruits, I made them the majority of my diet. I feel the difference when I haven't had enough lifeforce foods. If this is the first time hearing about food being lifeforce, try and look at these particular foods from an energetic, lifeforce level and make sure to eat enough of them every day, and then see how you feel.

Food is lifeforce which means that food is also vibration. High lifeforce foods like fruit, vegetables, and sprouted foods are high vibrational foods. Low lifeforce foods like meat, dairy, eggs, overcooked foods, and fried and processed foods, are low vibrational, so just imagine what food does to our vibration!

From quite early on during my second pregnancy I made a point to sit in the Sun with my belly out, whenever it was sunny. I wasn't sure what to expect but I know that baby loved it too. Every time I sat in the Sun he'd burrow forwards towards my belly button and became super active. He was completely aware of what I was doing.

For a long time, the Sun has been promoted as being dangerous, but in recent years, vitamin D deficiencies are becoming more and more common. If we build up our time in the Sun and be sun-smart, the Sun actually enhances our health, wellbeing, and spirituality.

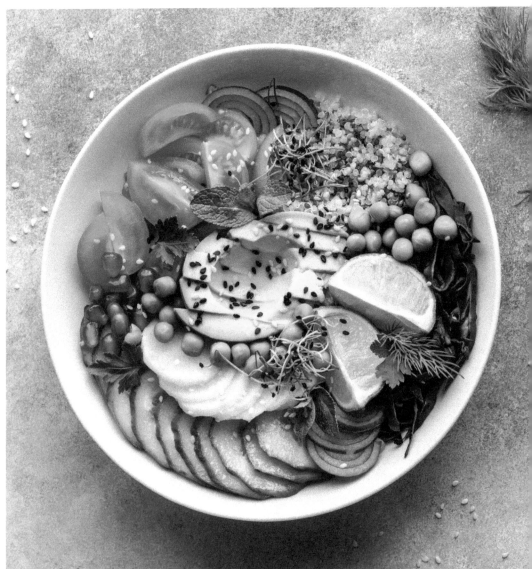

FOOD IS VIBRATION.

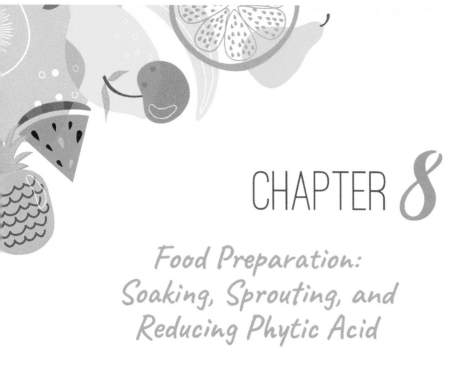

CHAPTER 8

Food Preparation: Soaking, Sprouting, and Reducing Phytic Acid

While eating nutrient-rich foods it is also vital to remember vitamin and mineral inhibitors and enhancers. The most common nutrient enhancers are vitamin D; eating your nutrient-dense meal while sitting in the Sun is perfect. Vitamin C is also a nutrient enhancer, with the exception of selenium and copper.

Eating foods that are rich in vitamin C, such as kiwifruit, oranges, capsicum, kale, tomatoes, and berries alongside your meals, will assist vitamin and mineral absorption. As mentioned previously, adding a 'good fat' to every meal also helps absorption.

One note to keep in mind is the number of nutrients that are lost during cooking, which is why it is important to eat raw vegetables or fruits alongside a cooked meal. Studies have shown that about 30% - 40% of minerals are lost during cooking; boiling, frying, parching and stewing showed the most mineral loss. When foods are boiled, the minerals end up in the water, which is later tipped down the sink. One way to decrease the number of minerals lost is to eat the boiled food with the leftover soup/stock. I like to pour it in a mug and drink once cooled. You can also add salt to the food before boiling, and boil the food with the lid on the pot which helps stop the minerals from escaping in the steam.

With vitamins, all methods except for pressure-cooking, steaming and in some instances, stir-frying, showed significant losses of vitamin C, B-vitamins, as well as antioxidants, chlorophyll, and soluble proteins. Steaming broccoli showed the best retention of nutrients; however, there is still some vitamin loss (22% - 34% loss). Pressure-cooked vegetables retained about 90% of their vitamin content; however, different cooking times will vary the result. When food pairing to enhance nutrients, bear in mind that certain cooked foods aren't the best sources, so food pair with raw foods, if possible.

The most common nutrient inhibitors are alcohol, coffee, caffeine, antibiotics, high levels of protein (inhibits calcium, magnesium and B-complex absorption), processed foods, fried foods, gluten, smoking, refined sugars, and the controversial, phytic acid.

Phytic acid is a natural substance that is found in grains, legumes, nuts and seeds. It is the major storage form of phosphorous in these plants. Phytic acid is known as a nutrient inhibitor which chelates micronutrients and prevents them from being bioavailable. This is because we lack enough of the enzyme *phytase* in our digestive tract to break it down. Phytase is an enzyme that breaks down phytic acid making it easier for the body to absorb nutrients. Without enough phytase in the digestive system, phytic acid becomes a mineral magnet. This means that the minerals eaten alongside phytic acid bind with the phytic acid, and then the minerals are excreted, rather than absorbed. Several studies have shown that phytic acid inhibits the absorption of iron, zinc, calcium, magnesium and manganese.

I'm not suggesting giving up phytic-acid-containing foods. Legumes, nuts and some grains in particular, are a staple in my house, but what the Western world has forgotten is how to prepare these foods properly. While soaking and activating nuts is becoming more and more common (which is also the best method to reduce phytic acid and release more nutrients within the nuts), grains and legumes are often overlooked.

Many Asian and Middle Eastern cultures have been soaking legumes and grains for hundreds of years. The best way to do this is to soak them in salt-treated water for one to two days before rinsing and thoroughly cooking. Soaking legumes and grains heavily reduces their phytic acid content, and I recommend soaking all legumes and grains before use. Furthermore, when cooking legumes, adding a bay leaf, or a half teaspoon of cumin, or kombu to the pot, will help digestion.

Low levels of phytic acid have been reported to have some beneficial effects on the body, so the point here is to reduce phytic acid by preparing these foods properly, especially if you have poor gut health or digestive issues.

Oxalate is another mineral inhibitor. Oxalate helps plants to get rid of extra calcium. In this sense, oxalate is fantastic for plants, but not so much for us because it inhibits our calcium absorption. Also, some people must eat a low-oxalate diet due to their higher risks of getting kidney stones. It is ideal to be mindful of your oxalate intake, especially if you rely on greens for your calcium. Eat high-oxalate foods like spinach, swiss chard/silverbeet, rhubarb, beans, and some nuts every now and then, and eat low-oxalate greens such as kale, romaine (cos) and other lettuces more often. Lentils and chickpeas also contain lower levels of oxalate.

Lectins are also known as nutrient inhibitors and are inflammatory molecules which can set off autoimmune responses. Lectins are carbohydrate-binding proteins present in most plants, which stick to the cell membranes in the digestive tract. Grains, legumes, seeds and nuts are essentially the 'baby' of that plant, and these proteins act as the plant's defense system. Much like the shell of a chicken's egg, the shell protects the 'baby' inside, just like lectins protect the 'baby' inside the hard outer casing of the lentil.

Lectins can cause digestive upset if the food is eaten raw or hasn't been prepared properly; however, not all lectins are the same. Some lectins are toxic, while others are beneficial. Always prepare these foods properly including soaking and sprouting legumes and wholegrains, and activating nuts and seeds. This combats both phytic acid and lectins. With nightshades, cook them and/or remove the seeds, and never eat raw potatoes. If nightshade vegetables still upset your body, remove them from your diet and try improving your gut-health. Nightshades can cause Restless Leg Syndrome (RLS) in some people, so be mindful of this if you suffer from RLS. Keep a food diary and add smaller amounts of nightshades back to your diet, if you choose to.

As a species, I do believe that we overconsume many foods, especially seeds. If you look at chia seeds it can take an entire adult chia plant to gain one tablespoon of chia; yet in the kitchen, one tablespoon of chia seeds doesn't go very far. Many seeds are also difficult to activate. With that in mind, I do believe that it's important to be mindful of our seed intake. The exception is hemp seeds, which are one of the only seeds without phytic acid and are low in lectins. From an Herbalism point-of-view, this is nature delivering the perfect seed for eating.

Nature has designed seeds to survive the digestive tract, which is why they are tough to digest. A plant's survival depends on its seeds being spread. Many plants purposely grow fruits that are bright and give off an irresistible aroma. This is to tempt an animal to eat it. The fruit is then digested but the seeds survive the digestion process and are later excreted. And this is where the plant regrows.

When you get into the groove of soaking legumes, you can sprout them too! Sprouted legumes are a powerhouse nutrient-dense food, and they also come to life, making them the perfect lifeforce foods - just like raw fruits and vegetables. Legumes and grains are dormant and contain zero lifeforce until they are sprouted, and lifeforce is one of the major keys to health and wellness.

My favourite sprouted legumes are lentils and mung beans. Both of these can be eaten raw, and I use them in salads, or turn them into hummus, or sprouted burger patties, which are lightly pan-fried. I've included my recipe at the end of the book.

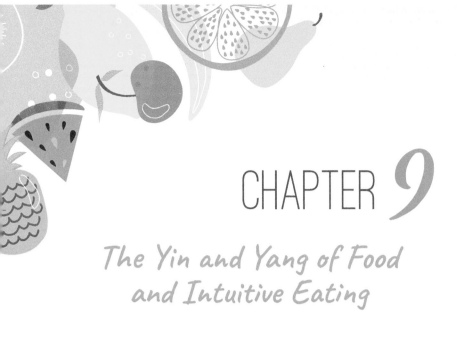

CHAPTER 9

The Yin and Yang of Food and Intuitive Eating

Many of you know about the benefits of raw foods. Eating an array of raw foods provides essential vitamins, minerals, carbs, proteins, lipids, enzymes, and phytonutrients. However, after cooking many of these foods, some of their nutritional value is lost. Bear in mind that cooked foods lose about 30% - 40% of the nutrients, which is better than losing all of them, so it is important to eat a mixture of both. This is because some foods must be cooked, such as potatoes and cruciferous vegetables. Interestingly, some food's nutrients increase after being cooked. For example, beta carotene increases in carrots and becomes more readily available once they are cooked. In addition, carrots become easier to digest. Also, many spices activate once they are heated.

Raw foods are considered 'yin' foods because they have a cooling effect on the body, and cooked foods are considered 'yang' foods because they have a warming effect on the body. Eating too many of one side disrupts the digestive fire, meaning that it weakens the digestive system. We should balance our yin and yang foods, with consideration of the climate that we live in.

If you live in a tropical climate, then more yin or cooling foods are better suited to 'cool' your body. And if we look at tropical climates, there is usually an abundance of fruit, paired with coconuts to keep us hydrated!

The opposite can be said for those who live in colder climates. In colder climates, tropical fruits do not thrive, but warming foods do, such as root vegetables and cruciferous vegetables, making it better suited to eat more warming foods in colder climates.

If you live in both climates, like we do in Australia, where it's super hot in summer and cold in winter, then it's important to eat with the seasons. One of the hardest foods we can eat during winter and when our bodies are cold are frozen foods. While I maintain my smoothies during winter, I get around this by using ingredients that have been kept at room temperature. I keep fruit on the bench top. If we are truly listening to our bodies, our bodies don't usually want cold foods during winter and instead crave hot and heavier foods to warm us, which helps us store energy. Our bodies use more energy trying to stay warm, which is why we're often hungrier and crave heavier foods in colder weather.

If we eat cold food while we're cold, our bodies have to work overtime to digest and warm up the food as well as our organs. For example, the spleen is a 'yin' (cold) organ and prefers 'warming' foods. So too many cold foods, especially when our bodies are cold, can deplete the spleen's 'fire.'

While this is considered the Yin and Yang of foods, it is also part of intuitive eating. Intuitive eating means listening to our bodies, to our intuition, when it comes to what and when to eat. Basically, eat when we're hungry; eat cooling and cold foods when it's hot; eat warming and cooked foods when it's cold. If suddenly you feel like mango, then eat it. This is your body's way of saying, "I need nutrients that are found in mangoes!"

You may have noticed that some vegan influencers have reverted back to an omnivore diet, or completely changed what they previously promoted to be healthy. This is because they've eaten what they thought to be healthy without proper knowledge of nutrition, hence it is dangerous to listen to influencers who do not have a nutritional background. Eating a lot of fruit and raw foods is amazing for the body, especially when healing an illness, but too many of these cooling foods without eating warming foods, causes an imbalance, which weakens the digestive fire. Once the digestive fire is compromised, the immune system suffers, and illness begins.

This also leads to the *Doctrine of Signatures*. The Doctrine of Signatures states that herbs and foods resembling various parts of the body can help target or treat ailments associated with those body parts.

For instance, walnuts look like a brain: left and right hemispheres, upper cerebrums and lower cerebrums, even the folds in the nut are just like the neocortex. We now know that walnuts help develop over thirty-six neurotransmitters for brain function.

Avocados and pears resemble the womb, and both target the health and function of the womb and cervix. Funnily enough, it takes nine months to grow an avocado from blossom to ripened fruit!

There are many other examples of the Doctrine of Signatures and how foods that resemble body parts are the areas that the foods target:

- Sliced carrots look like an eye, and science now shows that carrots enhance blood flow to the eyes.

- A tomato typically has four chambers and is red. The heart is red and has four chambers. Research shows that tomatoes are indeed heart and blood food.

- Kidney beans look like human kidneys and they help maintain kidney function.

- Dates, when sliced and opened resemble female genitalia, and for centuries, dates have been known to help the vagina, particularly the cervix.

- Celery, bok choy, and rhubarb, when the leaves have been chopped off, look like bones, and these foods target bone strength. Bones are 23% sodium and these foods are 23% sodium. If you don't have enough sodium in your diet, then the body pulls it from the bones, making them weak. These foods replenish the skeletal needs of the body.

- Sweet potatoes look like the pancreas, the organ which makes the hormone, *insulin*, and balances the glycemic index (GI) in diabetics.

- Peanuts look like testicles and have a profound effect on the testicles and male libido. Most people don't realize that *arginine,* the main component in Viagra, comes from peanuts!

- Grapefruit, oranges, and citrus fruits, when sliced open, look like the mammary glands. These fruits assist in the health of the breasts and the movement of lymph in and out of the breasts.

These are just several food examples of the Doctrine of Signatures. Herbs are also part of this and Herbalists have been using this method for centuries, long before science caught up with the healing powers of herbs and food.

Pears, bok choy, and oranges were just three of my cravings during my second and third trimesters. Pears aren't usually a fruit that I would normally eat, so when I began craving pears, I knew it was my body asking for the nutrients that pears provide.

There is a difference between *intuitive eating* and *cravings*. While we crave what we're lacking nutritionally and what our bodies need, we can crave what food is floating around in our blood. This is often the reason why some people go on a detox diet and then they suddenly crave a pie or cake. This isn't because their body needs substances from those foods, but during a detoxification period, the body releases toxins that were stored in the fat cells. When those toxins/ foods have been released and are floating around in the blood again, this can manifest as a 'craving.'

Intuitive eating is knowing our bodies and listening to our body's needs. Although we might not like to admit it, our bodies won't crave cake or pie. But we know our bodies will crave fruits and vegetables, raw/cold foods when we're hot, and cooked foods when we're cold. Intuitive eating also means eating when we're hungry rather than at allocated times, or at times of boredom.

CHAPTER *10*

The Link Between Certain Foods and Painful Breastfeeding

Is painful breastfeeding really a symptom of the food we eat? Various issues arise during breastfeeding, the most common being mastitis. Mastitis is diagnosed when a breastfeeding mama experiences inflammation of the breast associated with systemic symptoms. It is important to remember that our bodies are extraordinary vessels that operate wonderfully, if fuelled correctly.

The mammary gland is a magnificent organ. Colostrum lacks nutrients but is loaded with antibodies. These antibodies protect baby for the first six months of life. As baby suckles, there is some reflux, backward flow, into the milk ducts of the mammary gland. Should baby develop an infection, the organisms causing the infection are included in this reflux. Typically, by the next time baby suckles, the mammary gland will have produced the specific antibodies to help baby heal. Our bodies are astonishing!

One of the most common causes of painful breastfeeding is fungal infection due to yeast overgrowth. This is why I believe that it is crucial to watch your yeast intake, not only during pregnancy but in everyday life as well. Yeast overgrowth, specifically Candida, is one of the major underlying causes of dandruff, eczema, athlete's foot, acne, keratosis pilaris, toenail infections, candida-related insomnia, vaginitis, inflammation of the sinuses and/or ears, recurring urinary and vaginal infections, digestive disorders, oral thrush, mood swings, hormonal imbalance, and brain fog. All of these symptoms typically indicate a yeast overgrowth and fungal infection within the body. For breastfeeding mamas, the effect is that the fungal infection can spread through the mammary glands causing breast and nipple thrush, which can be extremely painful.

Symptoms of breast and nipple thrush can range from mild to severe stabbing pains behind the nipple, burning sensations in the breasts, and/or shiny, itchy or flaky skin on the areola or nipple. These symptoms are similar to vasospasms which I will address further on in this chapter.

Unfortunately, baby can then catch the infection from the nipple which leaves baby with oral thrush. Indications that baby has thrush include white patches in the mouth, which can look like milk curds, and on baby's tongue, gums or inside baby's mouth. Fussiness during feeding time due to pain in the mouth is another indication. Nappy (diaper) rash can be caused by many reasons, but it can also be an indication that the infection has spread through baby's digestive system.

Some GPs miss this diagnosis because they solely rely on checking for white patches on baby's tongue. Candida overgrowth and a fungal infection in the nipple don't always physically manifest in the breast or in baby's mouth. When the areola is itchy and appears red and/or crusty, the diagnosis may have been too quick without looking at other causes. This has resulted in many practitioners misdiagnosing mamas with dermatitis or eczema of the nipple; however, as mentioned at the start of this chapter, eczema and dermatitis are both typically underlying symptoms of a fungal infection. While there has been some controversy about whether it is *Staphylococcus aureus* (bacteria) or Candida (fungal) that causes burning nipple pain and breast pain, Candida has been proven to cause these symptoms as well.

As the yeast grows and spreads it leaves behind dangerous toxins which are essentially the yeast's waste by-products, *gliotoxins* and *acetaldehyde*. These toxic waste by-products have been linked to a wide range of disorders, such as depression and anxiety, brain fog, fatigue, nutritional deficiency, autoimmune conditions, systemic inflammation, and weakened immunity. Studies have also shown that gliotoxin is exceptionally high in patients with multiple sclerosis, an autoimmune disease affecting the central nervous system. As the Candida grows stronger, it forms a biofilm, a 'protective matrix' around itself, which increases the production of gliotoxin.

At smaller and proper levels, Candida is beneficial to the body and aids nutrient absorption and digestion. The beneficial bacteria in the body should typically keep Candida levels under control. However, if healthy bacteria levels are corrupted or if the immune system is compromised, Candida can overproduce and overgrow. This is where food choices are incredibly important because what we eat either fuels or inhibits Candida growth.

Whether you have overgrowth symptoms or not, it is always best to limit added yeast and Candida-feeding foods.

What feeds Candida? Candida is a yeast, a type of fungus, that is acidic in nature. Yeast feeds on sugar, so it is advisable to limit or cut-out refined sugars, refined carbohydrates, gluten grains, and grain starches. Additionally, it is advised to restrict yeast consumption, such as yeasty-refined-carbohydrate-bread and kombucha. Candida-overgrowth-suffers have also shown improvement by limiting mouldy foods, such as long-life shelf products, fruits that are susceptible to mould including fresh strawberries and blueberries when left at room temperature, peanuts, peanut butter, jams, and processed foods, especially those that contain citric acid.

Contrary to popular belief, the citric acid that is used in most commercially processed food isn't citric acid that has been derived from oranges or lemons. It is derived from a GMO black mold, *Aspergillus niger*, and is commonly found in spoiled produce. In 1917, a food chemist discovered that citric acid could be made from this mold, and it wasn't long before Pfizer began industrial-level production of citric acid. The mold is filtered, treated with calcium hydroxide to yield calcium citrate, then treated with sulfuric acid, which leads to the formation of citric acid. While many say that this form of citric acid is safe, many are intolerant and have allergic reactions to it.

Aspergillus niger has also been associated with otomycosis (fungal ear infection), cutaneous infection (fungal infection of the skin, hair or nails) and pulmonary diseases (a group of lung diseases such as emphysema, chronic bronchitis, and chronic asthma). Even though the mold has been treated, it may still cause issues. If you have candida overgrowth or are sensitive to mold, limit or cut out your commercial citric acid intake. Citric acid is found in many shelf products and long-life products, so realistically, limiting this form of citric acid is a good thing. If only citric acid was as simple as lemon juice!

Alongside fresh leafy greens and green vegetables, other foods to combat Candida overgrowth include sauerkraut and other fermented vegetables, raw coconut oil, apricots, flaxseeds, and turmeric. Green vegetables help alkalize the body which combats Candida's acidic nature, so eating plenty of greens helps too. If adding raw greens to a smoothie, chew the smoothie or swish it around in your mouth. This is to promote saliva production which prepares the gut for digestion. Limiting acidic foods, such as unsprouted or unsoaked grains, and heavily processed foods will also aid recovery.

You know my mantra, **prevention over cure**, so please remember to adjust your diet, so the yeast doesn't have a chance to overgrow.

Another complaint about painful breastfeeding is caused by vasospasms. Vasospasms happen when blood vessels tighten and go into spasm, causing the blood not to flow properly. Mamas with vasospasm of the nipple feel sharp pains and/or burning or stinging in the nipple, which is usually accompanied by sudden whitening of the nipple, and a colour change from red to blue, before turning back to its original colour.

Women who are more prone to nipple vasospasms tend to have cold hands or feet or poor circulation, low body mass index, and/or *Raynaud's phenomenon* in their family history. Mama may feel intense nipple pain which is worse when she is cold, or when the nipple is exposed to cold air. Some mamas describe the pain as burning, sharp, and throbbing. Avoiding known triggers will help to reduce nipple vasospasm, such as poor attachment to the breast and exposure to cold. Adding foods to the diet that promotes circulation will help too, such as oranges, ginger, goji berries, watermelon, sunflower seeds, and Ginkgo biloba. Ginkgo biloba promotes circulation and assists the immune system. Ginkgo biloba can be taken in small doses while pregnant and breastfeeding. Please see your practitioner before taking Ginkgo biloba for accurate dosage.

One of my favourite B vitamins, vitamin B6 (pyridoxine), and magnesium have been used to help alleviate nipple vasospasms (refer to Chapter 3 and 4 for food suggestions.) Vitamin B6 has been used to treat Raynaud's phenomenon, a condition in which the smaller arteries that supply blood to the skin constrict excessively in response to cold, limiting blood supply to the affected area.

How can you tell the difference between nipple vasospasms and Candida-related breast pain? The pain clinically associated with Candida infection is persistent, ranging from mild to severe, and is not relieved by the use of nipple shields, expressing, or applying heat. When the pain is relieved by heat, vasospasm is the likely cause. When the pain is related directly to infant feeding, the cause is likely to be mechanical.

Above all, with pain comes inflammation, and adding anti-inflammatory foods and limiting or removing inflammatory foods will also help alleviate pain. I will discuss this in the next chapter.

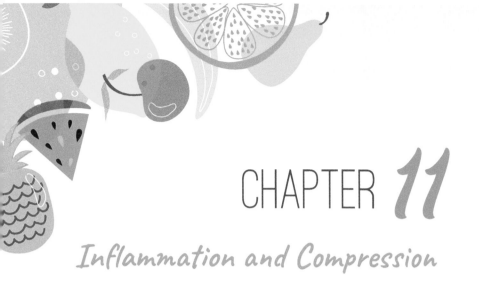

CHAPTER *11*

Inflammation and Compression

At the source of most pain is inflammation and/or compression, and limiting pain during pregnancy is crucial. Mamas should be happy, healthy, and as pain-free as possible!

Inflammation is the body's natural response to protect itself against harm and is essential in the healing process. There are two types of inflammation: acute and chronic. Acute inflammation, part of the immune response, is the body's immediate reaction to injury or assault due to physical trauma, infection, stress, or a combination of all three. Acute inflammation helps to prevent further injury and facilitates the healing and recovery process.

As soon as injury or pain occurs, the immune system dispatches an army of white blood cells to surround and protect the area. This results in visible redness and swelling. The same process happens if you have an infection. Acute inflammation tells us that something isn't right, and without it, simple infections could be deadly.

Chronic inflammation is the result of long-term inflammation and can also occur in response to other unwanted substances in the body, such as toxins or pathogens. Chronic inflammation can result in other diseases but isn't typically what causes pregnancy aches and pains.

If you are experiencing joint or muscle pain only during pregnancy, there is typically an inflamed or compressed joint or muscle. Lower back and hip pain are the most common complaints amongst mamas-to-be, and acute inflammation is a symptom. To help curb acute inflammation pain, limit or better yet, cut out inflammatory foods such as gluten, processed foods, fried foods, white bread and pasta, sodas and sugary beverages, margarine and trans-fats, and processed snack foods like potato chips and crackers. Also, adding anti-inflammatory foods such as celery, beets, pineapple, raw olive oil, raw tomatoes, almonds, berries, green leafy vegetables, and oranges to your meal plan will help. You can also add foods such as turmeric, turmeric tea, ginger, and ginger tea, but take these foods in much smaller doses because they are herbs, and safe herbs should be taken in smaller amounts during pregnancy.

Note: *Turmeric is activated once heated, and because it is fat-soluble, it is best served with good fats. Black pepper also helps activation.*

Adding more Omega-3 will also help. My absolute favourite sources of Omega-3 are avocados and hemp seeds. Hemp seeds are one of the only seeds without phytic acid and do not require soaking or activating. Hemp seeds contain decent amounts of all of the amino acids and they are a great source of calcium, magnesium, and potassium, amongst other essential nutrients. Flaxseeds and walnuts are also excellent sources of Omega-3.

Another cause of pregnancy aches and pains is compression. Compression occurs when the muscles or joints are pressed together. For example, sitting in a chair without activating the core, compresses the spine, which results in lower back pain. Fortunately, compression is easier to fix. Stretching the body, particularly the spine, and limiting exercises that compress the body, will help extend the body again. My personal favourite way to extend my body and relieve compression is yoga, which I will cover in Chapter 17.

Many mamas experience compression pain while sleeping. While it isn't always avoidable, there are a few things that mama can do to help alleviate it.

- Do lower back and hip stretches before going to bed. This helps to reset your body after a long day.
- Sleep with a pillow in between your knees or purchase a 'body pillow.' Body pillows have helped many mamas during pregnancy.
- If you sleep on your side, only sleep on your left side for digestive comfort and optimal blood flow.
- Or sleep 'diagonally' on your left. Sleeping on my left side, night after night, often left me with sore and compressed hips in the morning, so I slept diagonally. Lay on your left and place a pillow right behind your back, then lay back on the pillow. I found comfort in this position as my bodyweight was more evenly distributed, and I could stretch out my legs, one at a time. When my belly began getting quite large, I placed a pillow under my belly for support.

In any case, it isn't recommended to sleep on your belly, or flat on your back.

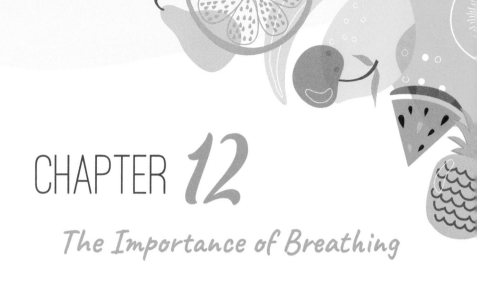

CHAPTER *12*

The Importance of Breathing

Proteins serve as a buffer, meaning that they help to prevent the pH of the body from getting too high, or too low. Our respiratory system helps balance our pH level as well. While it is common knowledge that the respiratory system is the breathing mechanism of the body, the respiratory system also maintains our pH level due to the exchange of oxygen and carbon dioxide. This exchange is performed by the lungs by eliminating carbon dioxide, a waste product given off by cellular respiration.

When we fail to breathe properly, we don't take in enough oxygen, and we don't exhale completely. This means carbon dioxide (CO_2) accumulates in our blood. High CO_2 levels decrease pH, leading to acidification of the blood, an acidic pH level.

When our breath is shallow we only half fill the lungs. When our breath is slow and deep, we completely fill the lungs and the diaphragm (also known as belly breathing), then we empty them completely. These deeper and slower breaths release more CO_2, which raises the body's pH level.

While it is easy to forget to breathe this way, every time you remember, try to breathe deeply.

You may have heard of Wim 'Iceman' Hof. He is well-known for his work on alkalizing the body by breathing properly. Experts doubted him; however, he also allowed scientists to use him as a test subject to test his theory. Everything that Iceman had publicized about breathing turned out to be true. Breathing properly does in fact alkalize the body's pH.

Our bodies have primary channels of detoxification: through our skin, through excretion, through our liver and kidneys, and through our lungs when we breathe. Deep breathing eliminates toxins from the body tissues and helps to improve the immune system.

You may notice when someone drinks alcohol that you can usually smell it on their skin and on their breath, no matter how much they've brushed their teeth. This is because the body is detoxing the alcohol from out of the body – through the primary channels of detoxification – the skin and the breath.

Energetically, inside of our systems is stale air, stale energy, air that resides inside of us for most of our lives if we have not breathed deeply enough. This is another reason why it is important to breathe properly; to exhale out the old stale energy and inhale new energy. Breathing deeply is also a form of meditation, which helps to relieve stress and is perfect for grounding and centering.

There are many different methods to breathe deeply, but below is my favourite one.

- Take some time out in a quiet place (or in a place where you can relax).
- Inhale through your nose (and fill up the diaphragm) for eight seconds.
- Hold your breath for four seconds.
- Then exhale out through your mouth for eight seconds.
- Repeat this process for several minutes, daily.

If you find eight seconds is too long, try inhaling and exhaling for four seconds, and then build up to eight seconds.

From baby's point-of-view, studies have shown that we have been cutting their umbilical cords far too early.

"In the womb, the lungs cannot take in air, so the baby doesn't inhale and exhale. The lungs are filled with fluid. Adults get oxygen from the lungs, but the fetus gets its oxygen from the umbilical cord. The two chambers of the infant heart beat at roughly the same interval, to bring oxygen from the umbilical region to the tissues and send it back again. At birth, this arrangement changes rapidly. The blood flow switches, so that now it fills the lungs. Now, here's the reason for concern: If you cut the cord before the infant clears its lungs, takes that first breath, and transitions its blood circulation to the lungs, you could deprive it of blood and oxygen—and also stress the heart." *<source www.nichd.nih.gov>*

I waited to cut the cord with Kaimana and the difference between him and Keilana was extremely obvious. Keilana, like many babies, vomited amniotic fluid not long after birth. With Kaimana, we waited to cut the cord and his lungs were clear. He didn't vomit at all!

Studies have also shown that babies who have experienced delayed cord cutting have 32% more blood by volume. Cord blood contains clotting factors that work with vitamin K, which is crucial to baby's health. Allow baby to gain this crucial cord blood before cutting the cord.

From a holistic point-of-view, it is also theorized that 'cutting the cord too early' is associated with why most of us don't breathe properly. Because the umbilical cord has been cut far too early, we never had a chance to breathe a deep and proper breath. Instead, our first breath was a half-breath, and this ailment stays with us for our entire lives. There is also a vast amount of lifeforce that flows from the placenta and into baby after birth.

Many doctors and midwives are now advising to wait before cutting the cord until the cord has stopped pulsating. This pulsating is clearing baby's lungs, delivering the crucial blood-clotting cord blood to baby, and pumping the placenta's lifeforce into baby. If this resonates with you, mention it to your OB/GYN, midwife, or doula and ask them to wait before cutting the umbilical cord.

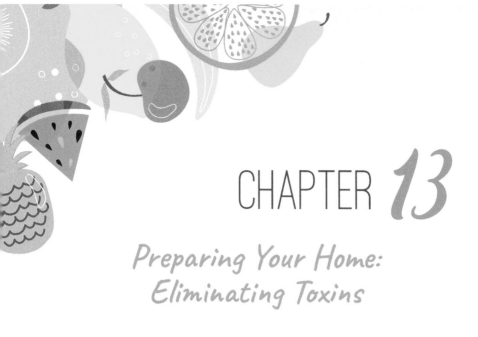

CHAPTER 13

Preparing Your Home: Eliminating Toxins

There are many toxins in our day-to-day lives. These toxins come from pollution, processed foods, sprayed foods, and from our cosmetics and household cleaners. However, there are other common toxins that many aren't aware of, and while it is difficult to avoid every single toxin out there, limiting exposure is key.

Tap water. Tap water contains many nasties, including chlorine and can include lead. If your tap water is fluoridated, then it also contains sodium fluoride and/or silicofluorides. These fluorides are toxic waste by-products of the phosphate fertilizer and aluminium industries. Natural fluoride is calcium fluoride and is found in spring water and soil. I don't recommend using plastic bottled water for environmental reasons and because microplastics have been known to leach into the water. I do recommend buying a water filter that can filter out all of the nasties. I'm a huge fan of the benchtop crockery filter systems. If you opt for a reverse osmosis filter, just be mindful that these filters take everything out of the water, including essential minerals and lifeforce.

Showers. Along with fluoride many local water supplies contain chlorine as well. When we have a hot shower the chlorine becomes a gas, and then we inhale it which leads to respiratory issues, sinusitis, skin and eye issues, and has also been linked to killing our good gut bacteria. Our digestive systems are designed to handle toxins, but our lungs aren't so robust. The pores of our skin open when we have a hot shower and the chlorine gas is absorbed directly through our skin and into our bodies. Unfortunately, shower fluoride filters aren't available yet, but there are shower filters that remove or neutralize the chlorine. The shower filter that I use is a vitamin C-based filter, which neutralizes the chlorine, and I did notice a massive difference after installing it.

Non-stick cookware. Polytetrafluoroethylene (PTFE) is the coating that makes products 'non-stick,' and it releases gases when heated. These gases have been linked to increasing our risks of developing cancer. Some non-stick cookware even comes with a warning to not use the cookware if you have a pet bird in the house! This just highlights the types of airborne toxins that this cookware releases. Try stoneware, ceramic, cast iron cookware, or PFOA and PTFE free cookware.

Microwaves. Microwaves are a form of Electro-Magnetic Radiation (EMR). When heating food in a microwave, the radiation that the microwave produces is absorbed by the water molecules in the food. This causes the molecules to vibrate which generates heat. While many say this food is completely safe, it has been reported that the eyes and testicles are vulnerable to the radiation emitted from the machine itself. While this is at higher levels of exposure, it is not recommended to stand in front of the microwave when it is operational. While studies haven't proven that microwaves are dangerous to humans, lethal effects of animal experimentation have been documented. I know it's super convenient to heat food in the microwave, but try ditching the microwave, and/or heating baby's milk in a glass bottle in hot water or a bottle warmer.

Electronic devices/Wifi. This is a bit controversial because so many people jump to the defense of technology. However, electronic devices all give off Electro-Magnetic Radiation (EMR). There have been several cancer and radiation experts that have warned against pregnant women using mobile phones and handheld devices because radiation can penetrate the placenta. I know it is harder to not use a handheld device these days, especially with work, but there are a few precautions that mamas can take.

- When using a handheld device make sure that there is an open window nearby.
- Sending text messages uses all of the phone's capability, so the EMR is at its highest. Try sending more instant messages or emails.
- If you use a Wifi modem at home, only turn it on when you are using the internet. Turn it off before you go to bed.
- Try not to be on your phone just before you go to sleep. Have at least an hour of time away from your phone/device before sleep. Particular frequencies and lights omitted from electronic devices mess with our REM sleep, our circadian rhythm, and melatonin - a chemical that helps regulate our sleep patterns. Studies have shown that melatonin was reduced by 50% in those who read with electronic devices. These levels also suggested that circadian rhythms had been delayed by about 1.5 hours.
- Use earphones, headphones, or the speaker function when talking on your phone, and limit putting the phone to your ear. Avoid wireless or bluetooth headphones.
- Never sleep with your phone near your head and turn it on 'airplane mode' while you sleep.

Baby monitors. Most modern baby monitors use FHSS or DECT technologies that operate on frequencies ranging from 1.89 GHz to 2.4 GHz. These are the same electromagnetic frequencies (EMF) that microwaves and WiFi routers use. There are legitimate concerns about the high levels of radiation that baby monitors emit.

Baby monitors, particularly ones with an ongoing video signal, continually send out strong bursts of radiation. These bursts can be sent out up to one-hundred times per second, even on standby mode. Baby's skull is thinner to allow for continued growth and brain development until about the age of twenty (when they are considered to be fully developed). A child's brain is extremely sensitive to electromagnetic radiation during these young years. Studies have shown that children absorb ten times more radiation than adults. If you need to use a baby monitor, opt for one that emits only low-band frequencies (35 to 50 MHz). These low-frequency monitors use analogue frequencies (like an FM radio) and do not pulse bursts of radiation. Also, do not place the monitor too close to baby.

BPA. Bisphenol A is in most plastics and in the lining of some food products, like canned foods and long-life milk and juices. BPA can leach into these foods, but what is also concerning is the use of hot foods in BPA containers. When the plastics are heated the chemicals leach out at about fifty-five times faster than normal. Purchase foods with BPA-free on the label and be mindful of takeaway food that comes in plastic. If you can, take your own metal, glass or ceramic containers in for the restaurant to fill.

Aluminium foil. Aluminium foil is generally safe to wrap food in, but where this differs is when it is used for cooking. The International Journal of Electrochemical Science asserts that aluminium can leach into the food, especially when used for acidic and spicy foods. When cooking with aluminium and a metal tray or pot, a short circuit has basically been created: aluminium (negative charge), and metal/stainless steel (positive charge), and then heat is added. This circuit charges the food that you are cooking, which then eats through the foil, especially if salt is involved, and you'll have tiny pieces of foil in your food. Opt for parchment paper and ceramic dishes and pots with lids.

Air fresheners and candles. Most air fresheners contain about 350 ingredients that aren't listed on the label including toxins like benzene, formaldehyde, and styrene. They're also made up of synthetic fragrances and substances. Many candles, especially cheap ones, are made from paraffin wax. This creates highly toxic benzene and toluene when burned, and these toxins, both known carcinogens, are the same as those found in diesel fumes. Opt for 100% soy, coconut, or hemp oil candles, and find a cleaner air freshener that uses essential oils.

Phthalates. Phthalates are a family of industrial chemicals that are used to soften plastic and used as solvents in cosmetics. Food packaging and many brands of disposable nappies (diapers) contain phthalates, as does anything that has been synthetically fragranced like perfume, moisturizers, deodorant, hairspray, soap, shampoo and conditioner, makeup, nail polish, and aftershave.

Phthalates are listed as a 'chemical of high concern' because of their endocrine disrupting effects, and according to studies, phthalates can also damage the thyroid, liver, kidneys, lungs, and reproductive system, particularly the developing testes. Phthalates can also cross the placenta and harm baby as well. Exposure during early pregnancy has been shown to alter hormone levels in baby, leading to male genitalia deformity, and affects baby's brain development as well.

Almost all plastic products, even some labelled as BPA-free, have been found to leach phthalates. Foods high in fat, like meat and cheeses, are more prone to chemical leaching.

Be mindful of purchasing food that is pre-wrapped in plastic, especially high-fat foods, and opt for cleaner cosmetics that do not add phthalates. There are plenty of options online and in the local health shops. If you prefer to wear perfume during pregnancy, spray your clothes at least ten minutes before wearing them, instead of spraying your body.

When it comes to nappies (diapers) not only do many disposable nappies contain harmful chemicals including phthalates, chlorine, dyes, and fragrances, they also take hundreds of years to break-down — eeeek! And these very nappies are also responsible for nappy rash in many babies. There are quite a few cloth nappy brands around now, plus there are a handful of companies who sell compostable disposable nappies that are free from the harmful chemicals.

Dioxins. Dioxins are a group of highly toxic environmental pollutants which are by-products of many industrial processes, such as chemical manufacturing, smelting, waste incineration, and chlorine bleaching of pulp and paper. Dioxins store in the fat tissues of animals, and it typically works its way up the food chain. While vegans are generally safe from dietary dioxins, these toxins are also found in disposable nappies as well.

Similar to phthalates, dioxins are highly toxic and cause damage to the reproductive, endocrine and immune systems, disrupts hormones, and is linked to cancer.

Mothballs. While mothballs aren't as popular as they were twenty years ago, the *naphthalene* found in mothballs can destroy red blood cells and has been proven to cause cancer in animals. Note, this has not yet been proven to cause cancer in humans.

Cosmetics also contain other nasties such as sodium laureth sulfate, bromate, cocamide diethanolamine, which is still added to natural products, and parabens. Opt for organic and eco-brands that do not contain these nasties. Be extra mindful of deodorant, particularly if you're using it on your armpits, as the mammary glands can extend into the armpits. Also, the milk-line runs along the armpits and you'll end up with deodorant chemicals in your milk.

It is crucial to be mindful of all baby products, as many contain a lot of nasties that should be illegal including baby formulas, cosmetics, and the food on the shelf in the baby aisle. Limit baby's exposure to plastic and opt for a glass bottle over plastic. If you haven't already, establish a 'no shoe policy' in your home. Baby is going to be crawling in no time, and we don't want baby crawling around on a floor that's had 'subway and public toilet shoes' walked through the house.

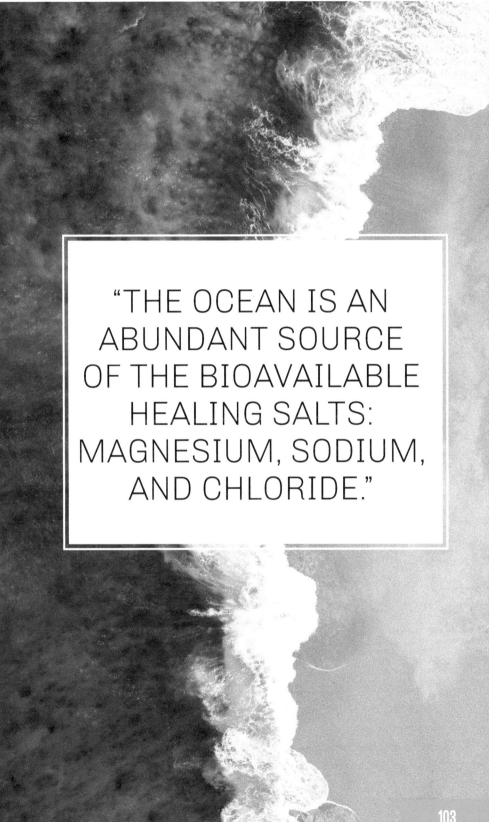

"THE OCEAN IS AN ABUNDANT SOURCE OF THE BIOAVAILABLE HEALING SALTS: MAGNESIUM, SODIUM, AND CHLORIDE."

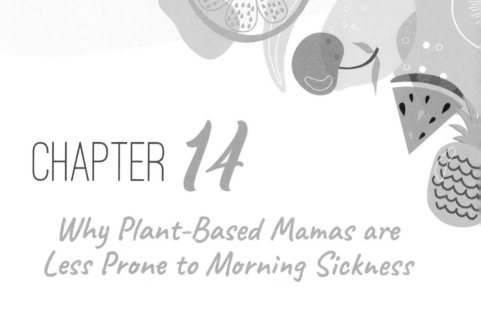

CHAPTER *14*

Why Plant-Based Mamas are Less Prone to Morning Sickness

For years, morning sickness has been blamed entirely on our hormones. While our hormones are affected by what we eat, there are a range of studies which conclude that morning sickness is our body's defense mechanism against pathogens and toxins.

Our bodies respond the same way when we get food poisoning, or if we've picked up a stomach bug. When a potential 'intruder' enters the body, our body's defense system does whatever it can to 'get the intruder out,' quick smart. This results in vomiting and/or diarrhea.

Food aversions during pregnancy are a tell-tale sign that our bodies are saying, "Hey, don't eat that!" Coincidentally, the most common food aversions by pregnant women are meat, fish, poultry, eggs, and dairy, followed by alcohol, coffee, and caffeinated beverages.

High saturated fat and animal protein intake are linked to morning sickness, an evolutionary sickness designed to protect baby, and mama, from pathogens. Our bodies instinctively know that animal proteins (meat, dairy, eggs) are high pathogen foods. When we eat pathogen-containing-foods or foods that may cause our body digestive stress, morning sickness is likely to follow. Foods that cause digestive distress are heavy gluten-foods, processed foods, trans-fats, and animal-saturated-fat foods. Our bodies know that these foods are tough on the digestive system, and like pathogen-containing foods, consuming them can also result in morning sickness.

Many pregnant women have aversions to alcoholic and non-alcoholic (mostly caffeinated) beverages and strong-tasting vegetables, especially during the first trimester. But the greatest aversions are to meats, fish, poultry, and eggs.

A study showed that animal products are dangerous to pregnant women and their embryos because they often contain parasites and pathogens. Pregnant women are often immunosuppressed, and as a result, pregnant women are more vulnerable to deadly infections. The scientists hypothesized that morning sickness causes women to avoid foods that might be dangerous to themselves and to their growing baby.

<source https://www.ncbi.nlm.nih.gov/pubmed/10858967 - Morning sickness: a mechanism for protecting mother and embryo.>

During my second pregnancy, I obviously didn't eat any animal products; however, conventional gluten also made me feel sick. I never ate a lot of gluten before pregnancy, but there were times when I was caught out and had no option but to eat a vegan dish which contained conventional gluten. While a lot of gluten products use bleached and pesticide flours, when I completely cut out conventional gluten products I never felt sick after that. Many mamas also acknowledge nausea and vomiting after eating gluten-containing foods.

My other food aversions were cumin and cooked garlic. Pre-pregnancy, I loved adding both to my dishes, but during my first and second trimesters, I couldn't stand the taste or smell of both herbs. For me, adding cumin to any meal ruined the dish, but adding garam masala or curry powder (both contain small amounts of cumin) was fine.

There were several instances when my husband cooked with garlic, and the mere smell of cooked garlic in the house made me feel nauseous.

However, my aversions to cooked garlic and cumin went away in my third trimester. My body was then ready for both herbs, so I added small amounts back to my diet.

There are conflicting studies about consuming cumin during pregnancy, but by the way that my body was responding, I couldn't deny that my body was telling me to steer clear of those foods or larger doses of those foods, during my first and second trimester. Food aversions are our bodies talking to us!

After this discovery, I linked this to alcohol consumption. When we drink alcohol our bodies go into 'instant detox mode' to eliminate this toxin from our body. When it comes to garlic, our bodies tend to react the same way, and no amount of teeth-brushing gets rid of the smell. This is because our bodies try to eliminate it the same way as alcohol: through the skin, and through the breath. Garlic, particularly raw garlic, has strong detoxing abilities which helps to remove toxins from the body. It is medicinal, so use in smaller amounts.

While Indian women have been eating many spices for hundreds of years (the safety of cumin has been debated because of this), it is known that eating too many spices results in 'smelly pores,' meaning that in larger amounts, the spices detox through the skin. My point is that any food that detoxes through the skin shouldn't be taken lightly.

If you have any food aversions, listen to your body!

CHAPTER 15

Should You Use Medicinal Plants and Herbs During Pregnancy?

Essential oils, herb oils, and therapeutic doses of herbs are heavily concentrated forms of the actual herb itself. This means that these substances can be dangerous when taken in concentrated doses. Typical cooking herbs and spices are safe in smaller doses, the amounts used in food, but excessive and concentrated amounts should be avoided. Some herbs should be avoided during pregnancy because they contain hormone-based constituents, or because they may result in harming the developing baby.

Many herbs contain chemicals that are structurally similar to two of the most important female hormones, oestradiol (an estrogen-based hormone) and progesterone, and may mimic them and interact with their receptors. Herbs with recognized estrogenic activity, such as sweet fennel and aniseed, may impact lactation if taken in larger doses.

The chemicals found in many common herbs can be transferred across the placenta and have the potential to directly affect the developing baby. These substances are called *teratogens* and may stimulate blood flow to the uterus, relax the uterine wall, or cause uterine contractions.

It is important to note that there have been very few studies on pregnant women and the effects of herbal remedies on the human embryo, primarily because it is exceedingly difficult to conduct ethical clinical experiments, so our knowledge is still developing.

However, based on the knowledge of the chemical makeups of certain herbs, and the affect that these herbs can have on women, the following is a list that should be avoided (but not limited to) during pregnancy.

- Aniseed
- Basil (safe in smaller amounts in food)
- Belladonna
- Black cohosh
- Black walnut
- Blue cohosh
- Boldo
- Borage
- Cedarwood
- Citronella oil (including the smoke from the candles)
- Clary Sage
- Clove
- Comfrey
- Dong Quai
- Ephedra
- Fennel
- Goldenseal
- Horseradish
- Hyssop
- Jasmine
- Juniper
- Licorice root
- Kava kava
- Marjoram
- Moringa bark
- Mugwort
- Mustard (safe in smaller amounts in food)

- Myrrh
- Parsley seed/oil/tea (the leaf is safe in smaller amounts in food)
- Passionflower
- Pau D'Arco
- Pennyroyal
- Peppermint oil (small amounts of tea is okay if no history of miscarriage)
- Rosemary (the leaf is safe in smaller amounts in food)
- Rue
- Sage
- Sassafras
- Savin
- Savoury
- Saw Palmetto
- Sweet Fennel
- Tansy
- Thuja
- Thyme (the leaf is safe in smaller amounts in food)
- Turmeric oil/large amounts of turmeric
- Valerian (only use as directed when pregnant as it decreases zinc levels in baby's brain)
- Wintergreen
- Wormseed
- Wormwood
- Yohimbe

Herbs used in cooking are generally safe, for example, you can add a small chunk of ginger to your smoothie, a bit of mustard to a dressing, or a handful of fresh thyme to your meal. Remember to avoid concentrated and high doses of any herb during pregnancy. It is also best to limit hot chillies and cayenne while pregnant as these foods can cause heartburn and acid reflux and are linked to morning sickness in some women. I have listed herbs for pregnancy, labour, and post-care in Chapter 21. Lastly, don't forget, if you experience any food aversions, no matter how weird they may seem, listen to your body!

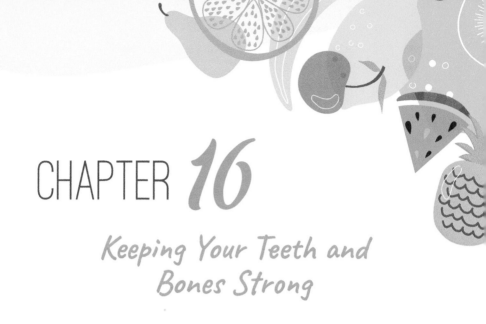

CHAPTER *16*

Keeping Your Teeth and Bones Strong

When we do not consume enough minerals for our everyday wellbeing, our body will release and use our crucial stores. This is when we begin to see concerning deficiencies. As previously mentioned, around 99% of our calcium stores are in our bones and teeth. If we're not consuming enough calcium in our diet, then our body will use our stores, leading to weaker teeth and bones, amongst other ailments.

All of baby's vitamins and minerals come from what we eat, and if we're not eating enough, baby will begin to use our stores. Baby knows exactly what to take, but problems will arise if there is little-to-nothing there for the taking.

These vitamins and minerals all work together to keep our teeth and bones strong and healthy.

Fat-soluble vitamins

Vitamin A. Vitamin A is often linked to good eyesight, but it also keeps the mucous membranes healthy and helps maintain salivary flow. Saliva is essential to teeth health as it contains minerals that strengthen the teeth, washes away bad bacteria, and keeps the mouth in a neutral or slightly alkaline state. If our saliva becomes acidic, it can result in tooth decay.

Vitamin D. Vitamin D is crucial for calcium absorption, and quite often, those with a calcium deficiency also do not get enough Sun. In the past, vitamin D deficiency has been associated with rickets.

Vitamin K. As well as being involved with blood clotting, vitamin K regulates blood calcium and is essentially a shield that helps block substances that break down the teeth and bones. It also helps our bodies produce *osteocalcin*, which is a protein (and a hormone) that supports bone strength. Without enough vitamin K2, our teeth become susceptible to tooth decay, as they lose the ability to defend against bacteria, to heal and to remineralize from the inside.

Water-soluble vitamin

Vitamin C. This vitamin helps to strengthen our gums and the soft tissue in our mouths. Bleeding gums is a symptom of scurvy, among other ailments, and vitamin C is used to treat it. Vitamin C can protect against gingivitis, the early stage of gum disease, and can prevent our teeth from loosening.

Minerals

Calcium. This impressive mineral helps build bones and provides structural support. In our mouths, calcium helps harden the enamel and strengthens the jawbone.

Magnesium. Magnesium is just as important as calcium. Around 60% - 65% of the magnesium in our bodies is stored in the teeth and bones. Magnesium supports and holds calcium and assists remineralization. It also stimulates the hormone *calcitonin*, which helps to preserve the bone structure by drawing calcium out of the blood and back into the bones. Osteoporosis has been linked to calcium deficiency, but also to magnesium deficiency as well.

CANDY MARX, MH, HHP

Potassium. Potassium improves bone mineral density. It also works with magnesium to prevent our blood from becoming too acidic, which can then leach calcium from our bones and teeth.

Copper. Copper plays an important role in bone development, and a deficiency is linked to brittle bones. Copper is also found in tooth enamel. It is essential for healthy teeth and bones.

Zinc. Zinc also plays an important role in bone health and healing. Increased amounts of zinc have been found at the sites of bone repair. Zinc also helps calcium absorption, and has been shown to fight against bacteria that causes tooth decay and is also found in tooth enamel.

Phosphorus. Like calcium and magnesium, phosphorus supports teeth and bone remineralization.

Sodium. As previously mentioned, our bones are 23% sodium which means that sodium is necessary for bone health.

Molybdenum. Molybdenum is abundantly found in our tooth enamel and helps form enamel.

What about fluoride?

As mentioned earlier, natural fluoride is calcium fluoride, and when we ingest calcium fluoride, the calcium helps to remove the fluoride from the body. Added fluorides, sodium fluoride and silicofluorides, which are added to tap water and most toothpastes, are not essential minerals. It is the calcium/calcium fluoride aspect that is important here.

Bleeding gums are a common ailment during pregnancy. To help reduce this, rinse your mouth out with salt water after brushing. Add pink Himalayan salt to a small glass of warm water and rinse thoroughly. The salt cleanses and kills bacteria within the mouth and helps remineralize the teeth.

It is also important to get into the habit of rinsing out your mouth with water after eating and drinking. This helps to protect the teeth from any sugars, acids, and bacteria.

While trying to get all of these nutrients into your diet may seem overwhelming, it's as simple as eating a wide variety of fresh fruit and vegetables, especially leafy greens, and a wide range of colours. As well as lesser soaked/activated nuts, legumes, seeds, and wholegrains. By eating a variety of foods, you will eat adequate essential vitamins and minerals, and 'essential supplement' with food-made supplements if and when you need to. For food sources, please refer back to Chapters 3, 4, and 6.

"The disconnect that exists between consuming a product and the reality it takes to bring that product to market is a phenomenon to itself. Animals are treated like commodities — referred to as property. We call it murder to kill a human being, yet create legal and illegal industries out of what would be regarded as torture if humans were involved. We pay people to do things to animals that none of us would engage in personally; just because we don't see it up close, doesn't mean we're not responsible.

Whether we are talking about factory farming, live export, animal testing, poaching, or the fur trade; logically, it's all on the same playing field to me. Suffering is suffering, murder is murder and the more helpless the victim, the more horrific the crime."

—DAMIEN MANDER

CEO/Founder of International Anti-Poaching Foundation,
Conservationist, Speaker, Former Navy Clearance
Diver and Special Operations Military Sniper
www.iapf.org

CHAPTER 17

Staying Active to Alleviate Aches and Increase Wellbeing

It is common knowledge that it's important to maintain an exercise regime throughout pregnancy to keep us fit for the big day, labour, but we also have to listen to our bodies.

During the first trimester, energy levels are usually a lot lower than during the remainder of pregnancy. A lot of women experience their worst bouts of morning sickness during this trimester as well. While your body is adjusting to the new changes, if you're tired and drained, take it easy and spend time outdoors, take a casual swim in the ocean, and work on your breathing. You have two more trimesters to start exercising again.

If you exercised regularly before pregnancy, keep it up and adjust your routine with your changing body. But, if you're like me and happen to have a retroverted uterus, going for long walks or doing anything high-impact is out of the question; especially during the first trimester before baby makes his way up, and off of the lower back. Gentle walks and swimming are advisable, and I highly recommend yoga as well. Yoga will keep your body stretched and extended, which will help alleviate muscle aches and pains, especially in the lower back and hip area because when these muscles tighten, the rest of the body is thrown off.

If you already do yoga, fantastic! Keep it up and adjust your practice with your growing belly. As the belly grows, the core weakens, so it's important to be mindful of that.

If you are new to yoga, I highly advise that you join a prenatal yoga class. If a class isn't local to you, then there are classes online. I only recommend doing online classes with a teacher who explains each pose and alignment properly. Getting the alignment correct is more important than how bendy you are. You may not notice the benefits straight away, but you will notice when you skip a few days. I've been practicing yoga for over eight years, and I still notice if I've skipped practice for more than two days. My lower back and hips always feel it, and one practice eases these ailments and stretches me out again.

Yoga not only stretches the body but there is an 'energy' side to each practice as well, which helps to push stale energy from out of the body. This is why yoga is perfect for stress relief. Also, being in practice helps to quiet the mind, promoting inner peace and mindfulness. Yoga is also a form of meditation which is extremely handy during labour. Meditation is a practice that should be done daily.

Stress manifests physically, so if we have no stress relief or time-out to ourselves, or somewhere to quiet our minds and reset, it can result in illness. A healthy body is very much connected to a healthy mind. And when mama is happy, baby is happy.

Our inner dialogue has a significant impact on our physical, mental, and spiritual health. If we tell ourselves that we're ugly, then we send ourselves 'ugly energy.' This, in turn, causes ripples throughout our energetic field, and contributes to the weakening of the immune system. The more ill-thoughts about ourselves, the weaker our immune system becomes. Our amazing bodies don't respond very well to negative thought patterns. When we tell ourselves that we're sick, we send ourselves 'sick energy,' but when we tell ourselves that we're healing, we send ourselves 'healing energy.' Next time you're feeling under the weather, try telling yourself, "I'm healing," instead of saying, "I'm sick." Our bodies are amazing, and it's important to remind ourselves of that. It's completely normal to have off-days, but never let a few off-days overshadow the rest of your amazingness!

And don't forget your Kegels! A strong pelvic floor gives you greater control of your pelvic muscles in preparation for labour and childbirth, and assists in recovery as well. If you happen to be one of the three-hundred women who suffer from Symphysis Pubis Diastasis (SPD), then Kegels will help this too. Eliminating inflammatory foods can also assist, and 'belly bands' relieve pelvis and lower back pain and pressure.

Pelvic tilts are another way to strengthen the pelvic floor and help relieve mild SPD pain. Instead of lying on the floor, lean against a wall and tilt your pelvis forwards and backwards, holding each tilt for at least three seconds. Whether you suffer from SPD or not, pelvic exercises should be added to your regime.

SPD occurs when the ligaments that connect the two halves of the pelvis soften. This occurs when the body releases the hormone, *relaxin*, which causes the ligaments in the pelvis to loosen. Generally, this is a good thing as it makes birth easier for mama and baby. However, sometimes the separation is exaggerated and can become quite painful for mama. Pubic bone and pelvic tenderness are normal, but it shouldn't be painful. If you do experience any pain, please see your OB/GYN or health practitioner.

Strong hips will also support recovery. Squats help strengthen the hips which can help alleviate pubic bone and hip tenderness. However, speak to your health practitioner first if you suffer from SPD.

A common but not very well-known condition that can arise after childbirth is *Diastasis recti*, or abdominal separation. It is more common in women who have carried a high birth-weight baby, a multiple pregnancy, or have had more than one pregnancy. If you still look pregnant weeks or even months after giving birth, you may have Diastasis recti. To check if you have it, lay on the floor with straight legs, tense your abdomen, and lift your head and upper body slightly. Place your fingers just above your belly button and see if you can push them through the abdomen. You should be able to feel the muscles on each side, and what you're looking for is the gap between those two muscles. Typically, a gap of 2.7cm or more means you have Diastasis recti.

There is a plethora of information online about how to heal it naturally, and, it's super important to give your body time to heal. Many mamas wait six weeks before they start running and doing sit-ups, but if you have separated abs, sit-ups makes it far worse.

Personally, after giving birth to Kaimana, I waited until my body was ready before my first (gentle) workout, which was eleven to twelve-weeks post-partum. But I didn't start exercising properly until twenty-weeks post-partum. When my body was ready, I went for a daily hour walk and implemented gentle exercises that helped strengthen my abdomen, hips and pelvis. Once my body felt ready, I started yoga again. Just remember that there's no rush to get back into shape! It took forty-or-so-weeks to grow baby, so be patient with your body returning back to normal. Always listen to your body!

How much weight should I gain during pregnancy? There is no number. We are all different. I have seen many mamas upset at themselves because their Doctor has told them that they've put on too much weight, even though it was mostly belly-weight. Don't fret if you've put on 10kgs and baby only weighs 1kg! Not only are you carrying and growing another human being inside of you, but the placenta itself weighs a few pounds, as does the amniotic fluid. We also gain extra weight in our breasts and our blood volume increases. While we typically have 4.5 - 5.5 litres of blood circulating the body, but during pregnancy we produce up to an extra 50% – an extra 2.5 litres of blood or so. We also store 3kg - 4kg of subcutaneous body fat (the fat under our skin) for breastfeeding. Unless you are unhealthy and severely overweight pre-pregnancy, don't worry too much about the weight that you gain during pregnancy. The weight mama carries is far more than just baby's weight.

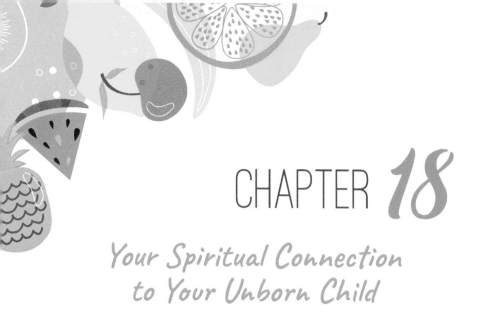

CHAPTER *18*

Your Spiritual Connection to Your Unborn Child

Do you believe babies randomly select us as their parents at conception? Like a lucky-dip, as in, we have no way of knowing who we're going to get until baby is born? Or at least until a scan tells us whether we're having a boy or a girl.

Or do you believe that our babies choose us long before conception? Perhaps way before we even decided to have kids?

I'm going to share my experiences with my two babies which will pretty much explain my beliefs on this topic.

I was in my late teens when I began to dream about a little girl. I could never see her face very clearly, but I felt her gentle soul around me. Fast forward a few years, I was only a week or two into my first pregnancy, and I just knew. I knew I was pregnant without being tested. At about four or five weeks along, I had the most vivid dream of this beautiful, gentle little girl with sandy-blonde-hair and light-coloured eyes. She would have been around three-years-old when I saw her, as she stood in front of me and held my hips. As I looked down towards her, she looked up at me and smiled, with her head tilted slightly to one side.

When I awoke, I knew who that little girl was. It was the little girl that I had encountered in my late teens, and I knew that this beautiful little girl had come to my husband and me.

Without being told or confirmed by scans, I was adamant that we were having a little girl, and that she would have fairer features, which is less likely for me due to my darker features. No one said I was crazy, but they were all shocked when a baby girl with fairer features was born.

When my daughter was around five or six-years-old, I began to dream about a little boy. I saw this little boy quite a few times. Sometimes he was a baby, other times he was a toddler, and a few times he was a teenager. Likewise, three of my family members dreamed about this little boy too, in different stages of his life, and they knew he was my son.

Skip forward a few years, I was literally only two or three days pregnant when I knew. And I also knew that the little boy from my dreams had arrived. As with my first pregnancy, I was just as adamant that I was carrying a boy this time around. Not just any boy, but the boy from my dreams.

I have no doubt in my mind that our babies choose their parents long before their parents even consider having children. From a soul level, we know who our children are going to be, but while we are here on Earth still trying to figure it all out, we forget about this connection. We forget that our family extends past our blood-line; our families extend into the spiritual realms of those who have passed and to those who are yet to come.

When you put this into perspective the connection between parents and our babies is unfathomable. These sweet little souls know exactly who we are, sometimes, before we even know who we are ourselves. While mama is carrying baby, baby is completely aware of what is going on. They know when mama is upset, they know when mama is stressed or angry or sad, and they know when mama is happy, healthy, and thriving. It's important to remember our connection to our babies and to tune into them. By this I mean, take some time out and use your intuition to talk to baby. You may surprise yourself by how much they can communicate with us while still growing inside of us!

Babies are amongst the highest vibrational beings on the planet, and every decision that we make effects that. They want to maintain their high vibrational state, and what we eat, where we go, who we surround ourselves with, what we think, and how we feel while we're pregnant, affects baby's vibration.

With my second pregnancy I was far more aware of what my baby was trying to tell me, and this time around, I listened. Due to work commitments or even being out to do the shopping, there were certain places, people, and foods that baby just didn't like.

He disliked being at the shopping mall, which I understand entirely because it's indoors with crowds of people who all have different kinds of energy. The energy builds up with nowhere to go, and like smoke when it has nowhere to go, it builds up and stays in the room.

I eventually started to realize that baby didn't like being in that particular environment because he'd burrow backwards towards my spine, and almost instantly I felt nauseous, drained, and tired. It felt as if I had walked for miles and my body ached, or that I had eaten something that I shouldn't have. However, as soon as I left the shopping mall and went outside into the fresh air, baby burrowed forward again, the nausea dissipated, and my body stopped aching.

Food aversions are our bodies telling us, "Hey, don't eat that!" but if you really think about it, baby has something to do with this too. Baby knows!

Scientists are beginning to understand the difference between nurtured children and unnurtured children. Well-loved and nurtured children's brains are wired differently to unnurtured children, which contributes to brain development and immunity strength. A well-loved and nurtured child will typically have a stronger immune system, be more intelligent, happier, and more affectionate than an unnurtured child.

Many women have asked me what I think about 'controlled crying'. To be honest, I don't agree with it, nor having a room separate to baby. I'm a huge fan of co-sleeping! When baby is born, baby is at his or her most vulnerable. Being born is a tough gig, and they need that 'safety net' to feel secure. They've been in mama's safe and cosy womb, and being 'outside' makes baby feel vulnerable. Newborns feel scared when they're left alone, and when they feel scared, they cry. When mama leaves the room, baby has no idea if she is coming back! Many mamas see the progress with their babies, as they tend to cry when mama leaves the room. But once they begin to understand that mama comes back and that mama is there when they need her, they begin to feel safe and nurtured. If we make them 'self-soothe' by crying themselves to sleep, they don't feel safe or nurtured, and their brains begin to wire differently.

Studies have shown that nurturing a child from birth helps them develop a larger hippocampus, the brain region important for learning, memory, and stress responses. Nurtured children typically do better in school and are more emotionally developed than unnurtured children. Brain images have shown that a mother's love physically affects the volume of her child's hippocampus. In this study, the nurtured children had hippocampus volumes that were 10% larger than children whose mothers were not nurturing.

Dr Joan Luby of the Washington University School of Medicine said, "We can now say with confidence that the psychosocial environment has a material impact on the way the human brain develops. It's put a very strong wind behind the sail of the idea that early nurturing of children positively affects their development."

We can learn by putting ourselves in baby's shoes. If you're completely bed-bound, vulnerable, and upset, how would you feel if your partner or parent walked into the room, touched your belly, and then walked out again? Or what if you were upset and no matter how much you cried, no one came to comfort you? What a lonely world that would be!

Babies also wake up crying because they need to be burped or need to clear mucous from their airways. Until baby can burp himself, he needs help. Lift baby up to your shoulder and rub his back; he will burp or spit-up if needed. A lot of the time baby will go straight back to sleep once the burp has been released. If practicing controlled crying, baby will be uncomfortable and sometimes in pain, if left unassisted.

Just like us, babies can also experience trauma, and while many say babies don't remember their infancy, trauma stays hidden within the body, in our DNA, and even in our bones. If baby has a traumatic birth or experiences any type of trauma or pain, those buried feelings and experiences stay suppressed in baby's body and may manifest later in life. It's crucial to be mindful of how baby enters the world, what happens to baby after birth, and how we raise baby. How we treat our babies either sets them up to feel secure and loved, or the complete opposite.

Spiritually, our babies chose us a long time before they came to Earth. They waited, and waited, and waited for that glorious day of conception. If we make our babies cry themselves to sleep, or segregate them into a separate bedroom, we become less and less of a 'spiritual and emotional rock,' and that connection between us and our babies begins to weaken. For many parents, this connection isn't important, mostly because they're unaware of it. However, nurturing our children is an important factor for their health, development, and happiness.

CHAPTER *19*

Using Nature to Cleanse

I'm a huge believer that the Earth and Sun provide us with everything we need. Trees and plants to give us shade, shelter, oxygen, clean the air, provide us with food and medicine, and an abundant eco-system that helps keep us alive. The Sun gives lifeforce, warmth, and solar energy. The ocean provides us with food, like sea vegetables, a diverse eco-system, salt water to heal us and cool us down, and also cleans the air. The ocean absorbs almost the same amount of carbon dioxide as plants! Animals all have their own purpose in helping keep the eco-system healthy and abundant.

All of these wondrous natural beauties help us cleanse as well! By this, I mean that nature helps us physically, mentally, and spiritually cleanse.

Let's start with earthing. Earthing is a technique where we stand or walk on the Earth, barefooted, either on grass or sand, or even dirt. By doing this, we come into direct contact with the Earth, the Earth's energy, and the Earth's electrons. These free electrons are taken up into the body and could be referred to as 'nature's antioxidants,' which help neutralize free radicals. The Earth is a conductor of free electrons and so are all lifeforms on the planet, including us.

Spiritually, earthing is also about connecting to the Earth, being mindful, present, and conscious, and acknowledging the gift of life that we have on this beautiful planet that we currently call home. Acknowledging 'Her' presence is also about giving thanks.

You may have noticed that many animals love to lay in the Sun, but if you've ever had the privilege of raising an animal or being in close contact, you may have noticed that animals 'earth' too!

As mentioned earlier in the book, the Sun is one of my favourite beings, who I call, *Father Sun*, to go with *Mother Earth*. The giver of lifeforce, essentially, the giver of life! Did you know that we can also use Sun energy to cleanse? You may have known that sunlight acts as a natural bleach and deodorizer. In fact, many people leave certain items or furniture in the Sun to get rid of marks and odours. Now, look at this same concept at an energetic level. Sun energy not only cleanses physical items, but it cleanses us energetically as well.

After my yoga practice, which I do outside in the Sun if weather permits, I like to sit in a half-lotus position facing the Sun, and 'feel' and 'visualize' the Sun's energy, streaming down like a bright golden ray into my body. Like earthing, sitting in the Sun is not only a natural cleanser, but a way to connect with and acknowledge 'His' presence and offer thanks.

The ocean offers powerful cleansing and healing properties. Salt is one of the most cleansing elements, both physically and energetically. Breathing in the salty air promotes healing for the respiratory system and for those with asthma, bronchitis, and sinus pressure. Many people swim in the ocean when they feel a cold or flu coming on, or when they don't feel too well. There have been times when I've felt flustered and the only way that I could relieve it was to swim in the ocean. Throwing on a snorkel and watching the peaceful lifeforms under the sea is a meditation on its own!

As previously mentioned, the ocean also helps alleviate aches and pains thanks to the natural healing salts: chloride, magnesium, and sodium.

Another way that we naturally detox is through the soles of our feet. Getting some Sun, Earth, and ocean water onto our soles assists this natural cleanse.

Spending time in nature is also good for the soul. Trees have such a powerful calming effect. Have you ever put your hand on a tree's trunk and purposely tried to feel its energy? Like earthing, this is also an energy exchange and a conscious interaction to say, "Hey, thank you! I love your work!" While all trees also clean the air, ferns in particular, let off probiotics. Just the simple act of walking through a forest and inhaling the smells of nature enriches our gut and beneficial bacteria. If you or your little ones have breathing issues, try placing a potted fern next to their bed, and add more indoor plants to your home.

Energy is frequency and vibration, and everything is energy. Plants and trees have their own frequency, which can be heard during deep meditation or using specific instruments. Imagine standing in a forest or in a field of sunflowers and hearing the choir of song that emanates from the plants. It's nothing short of miraculous. They can be heard using instruments, and although the frequencies cannot often be heard without them, our brains and hearts feel these high vibrational frequencies. We unconsciously hear their song all of the time. It's no wonder why we always feel better after spending time around trees and plants - in nature!

Spending time in nature, consciously acknowledging our surroundings, and being grateful, is cleansing, calming, and good for the soul. Whatever is good for the soul is good for mama and baby!

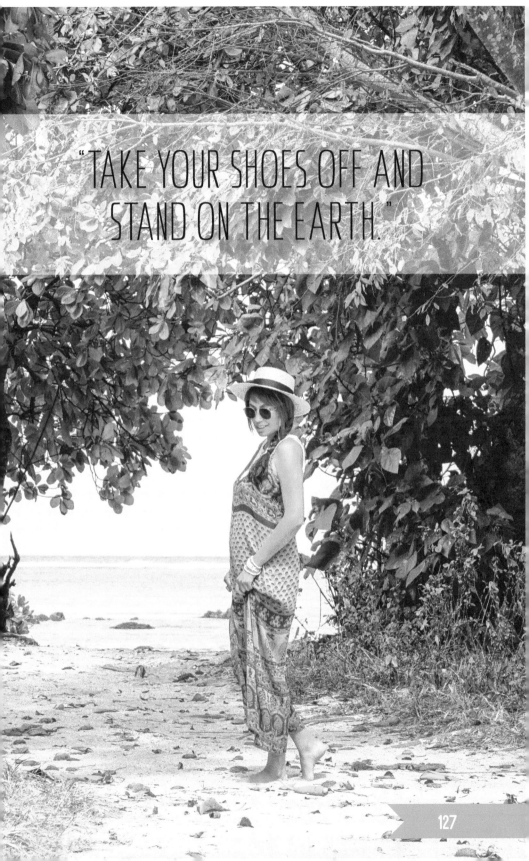

"TAKE YOUR SHOES OFF AND STAND ON THE EARTH."

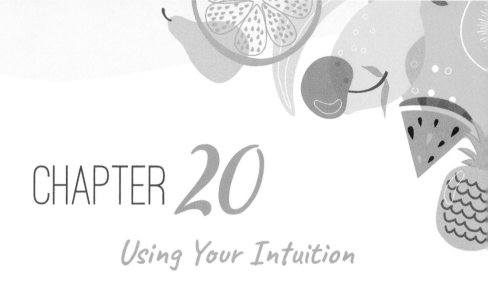

CHAPTER *20*

Using Your Intuition

Mama's intuition is one of the most important senses that we have. That gut feeling, or that feeling of 'just knowing' with no way of explaining it, except for "I feel it." Our intuition strengthens when we're pregnant and we should learn to listen to it.

It's easy to doubt ourselves. "What if I'm wrong?" That thought creeps into every single person's mind, more than once, but, we must learn to say, "What if I'm right?"

When we listen to ourselves our intuition strengthens, just like a muscle, so please mamas, when your 'gut' speaks to you, listen! If something feels right, follow that feeling. If something feels off, say so and speak up.

Our intuition comes in handy all of the time, especially during pregnancy and childbirth. Most mamas go into the delivery room with a birthing plan, and whether things go to plan or not, it's important to listen to what our intuition is saying.

For my first pregnancy, I went into the delivery room with unrealistic expectations. I say unrealistic because my antenatal (prenatal) class didn't truly prepare me for what was ahead. I understand that antenatal teachers don't want to scare mama, but not knowing the truth about what happens threw a curve ball at me, and my birthing plan went out of the window. My antenatal class taught me that contractions felt like period pain, and I thought to myself, "Yep, I can handle this without any drugs!" Oh boy, was I wrong. Because events didn't go as planned, I was pretty much outside of my comfort zone and felt extremely vulnerable during labour. My gut was telling me to stay upright during birth, but because it wasn't 'normal,' and, because I didn't feel as if I could speak up, I ended up lying on a bed. I used the gas, but when the contractions became super intense, I asked for the epidural. However, the epidural didn't work. Looking back at it now, I am glad that it didn't work because I was able to walk around not long afterwards, and I wasn't bed-bound. Once I knew what the pain was like, I knew that I could go drug-free for the birth of my second baby.

After Keilana was born, I noticed that no one asked for my permission when it came to who was in the room, and what happened to Keilana after birth. I had a group of students enter the room to watch me; I'm a private person and giving birth is a private moment. Giving birth in front of an audience was not at all ideal. The midwives also took Keilana away and poked and prodded her before I was allowed to hug her. In all honesty I wasn't prepared for them to make my decisions for me; I thought I'd be asked. I also didn't like that the partners are asked to leave when nightfall comes. How crazy is that? Mama has been through so much and can be super vulnerable, and asking mama's only support person to leave is ridiculous. It's a time for our partners to bond with their newborn child as well.

The second time around, I knew exactly what I was going to do differently. I knew that I had to use gravity, that I wanted to birth in water, and that I had to speak up and basically dictate what I wanted to happen. Unless you're having an epidural, it doesn't make sense to lay on a bed and push against gravity. Using gravity during labour has been done for thousands of years. Even the Ancient Egyptians used gravity, as many of their carvings show women squatting, kneeling, and using a birthing-chair during childbirth.

We want baby to come out as easy as possible, so why have we been lying down for all of these years?

Well, the origins are actually quite creepy. It is said that lying down during childbirth was popularized because King Louis XIV of France, enjoyed watching his wives and mistresses give birth. He had twenty-two children.

In the American Journal of Public Health, it says, "Since Louis XIV reportedly enjoyed watching women giving birth, he became frustrated by the obscured view of birth when it occurred on a birthing stool and promoted the new reclining position. The influence of the King's policy is unknown, although the behavior of royalty must have affected the populace to some degree. Prior to this time, the recorded history of birthing indicates upright birth postures were used extensively."

It is reported that when the lower classes learned that the king was a fan of the lying position, they too adopted the practice.

There have been a growing number of studies about 'directed pushing.' This term is also called 'Valsalva' pushing and is pushing without mama necessarily feeling the urge to push. Mama is instructed to inhale, to hold her breath and to maintain a steady pushing effort for approximately ten counts, three or four times through each contraction. Research does not support the widespread practice of directed pushing, which has been shown to stress the maternal cardiovascular system, reduce circulating oxygen, and trigger changes in the fetal heart rate. Directed pushing also brings on early exhaustion. Research also shows that mama should delay active pushing efforts until the body's natural urge to push is recognized. Essentially, directed pushing is not listening to your body, or to your intuition. When it's time to push, your body tells you! Whether you have a natural birth or not, always listen to yourself because your body will tell you what you need to do.

If you do opt for a natural birth and can birth without an epidural (it's hard, I know), then see how it feels to use a birthing bath. We are almost weightless in water, so kneeling or squatting in a bath is more gentle on the joints, and the warm water acts as a natural pain reliever. I gave birth to Kaimana in a birthing bath, and to me, water births are a game-changer. Being upright and being weightless make labour so much easier, and as soon as I jumped into the bath, the warm water was instantly soothing. There was also a slight suction force that helped Kaimana come out without intensely pushing. And, I was the first person to touch Kaimana which meant a lot to me, after my experience having Keilana.

If using medical help, make sure your midwife or OBGYN has experience in water-birthing as there are some precautions that must be taken. For example, when baby's head comes out, his head cannot leave the water and then go under water again. This means that mama must choose her birthing position carefully, as being on all-fours can mean that baby's head may accidentally leave the water and go under again. Also, mama can't get into the bath too soon as it can stop her contractions, and the water can become unsanitary. Watch online water-birthing videos where mama delivers her baby herself and it'll help you know what to do.

A lot of women ask me about home-birthing and if it is the best decision to make. The best decision to make is what feels right for you! Some women prefer home-births, some women prefer hospital births, and some women prefer free-birthing. All have advantages and disadvantages, but it's important to choose what's right for you and baby.

In Australia, a home-birth is expensive due to hiring a midwife or doula. I love that baby is born in a calm and peaceful environment that is familiar to mama, rather than in a chaotic hospital that can have a number of random health practitioners (and students) make an appearance in the room. However, hospital maternity care is free if you're a public patient. A few home-birth mamas have mentioned that they didn't like that their partner had to clean up the 'mess' afterwards. If complications do arise, then a hospital is the place that you want to be, but the majority of women who have a low-risk pregnancy have safely birthed at home. If you or your family have a history of losing a lot of blood during labour, then the hospital is the safer choice.

If you prefer a homebirth, make sure you're a low-risk pregnancy and find an experienced midwife or doula that you trust. Recommendations from other mamas will help too.

Free-birthing is when mama gives birth at home without a registered medical professional present. Mamas have been choosing this option because they didn't want to birth at a hospital, and/or they couldn't find a midwife who would do exactly what they wanted, or they couldn't afford one. The reason why mamas are opting to birth away from the hospital is generally because of their first experiences giving birth. They felt like they were pushed into things that they didn't want to do, with many mamas saying that they felt like they had no choice about what happened to their babies straight after birth.

Being born is a tough gig for mama and baby. By the time baby is born, baby has been through a lot! After being born, baby's umbilical cord is cut, then baby is injected and pricked, and in some countries medical professionals automatically administer *Erythromycin* antibiotics to babies eyes. Free-birthing mamas choose to give birth at home because all of that happens without mama's consent. In many cases, mama has tried to intervene, but some midwives have told mama that it was illegal to refuse! This, of course, is not true. The pressure placed on mamas and the antics to enforce it, are absurd.

Our bodies are amazing, and we are more than well-equipped to have baby without a medical professional present. Unfortunately, many professionals make mamas doubt their ability to naturally give birth, which I believe, takes mama's power – her mana, or inner strength. I have spoken to many mamas that felt like their doctor put unnecessary fear into them, and/or prematurely tried to intervene or schedule a c-section. Our bodies are spectacular vessels that are designed for this! With emergencies being an exception, don't doubt yourself as that doubt will effect your labour. Our mindset has everything to do with how we birth. Be in your power, remember your mana, and know that you got this!

If you're still unsure about home-birthing or free-birthing, have baby at a hospital, and write down a detailed birthing plan and give it to your midwives. Outline exactly what you want to have happen, and what you don't want to have happen. The hospital staff may make you feel like you have to do it their way, but you have the right to refuse. It's your body, your baby and your plan! It will also help to ask your partner to never let baby out of his/her sight, as some midwives have been known to rush baby away from mama straight after birth.

However, I do feel as if this is changing, because when I had Kaimana the midwives were fantastic. My main midwife was quite happy that I opted against painkillers, and when the pain became incredibly intense, she encouraged me to keep going. She also knew to delay the cord cutting, she didn't take Kaimana away from me, and she encouraged immediate skin-on-skin contact. She also delayed weighing Kaimana until I was ready to hand him over. My experience at the hospital with Kaimana was a lot more positive, compared to my experience at the hospital with Keilana.

Skin-on-skin contact with baby straight after birth, allowing baby to make eye contact with you and your partner, and leaving the umbilical cord attached until the cord or placenta stops pulsating are important. When you feel comfortable, then let the midwives weigh and measure baby. There's no rush in knowing baby's weight and length.

It's also become standard practice to inject synthetic *oxytocin* into mama straight after delivery, in an attempt to make the placenta expel quicker and to help the uterus contract. This injection wasn't around when I had Keilana, so it is a fairly new practice in Australia. Our bodies expel the placenta and our uterus' contract without this injection. Oxytocin is a hormone that our bodies release naturally during labour and when baby begins to breastfeed. Having the synthetic version injected into mama is only really necessary if mama is bleeding too heavily, as it helps to stop heavy bleeding, or if you can't breastfeed.

I suggest that you read up on what happens straight after birth, so you can make well-informed decisions. Also, chat with your practitioner about using baby's cord blood for newborn screen testing. Some practitioners are aware of this, but many aren't. And don't be afraid to speak up if something doesn't feel right.

As mentioned earlier in the book, sometimes mamas feel like their midwives or OB/GYN have a schedule to keep, so they pressure mama to be 'quicker' than what feels natural to her. In many cases, they do what's best for the hospital, instead of what's best for mama and baby. You and baby are on your own schedule, and it's important for you and your health practitioners to know that. Listen to yourself and listen to your intuition. You got this!

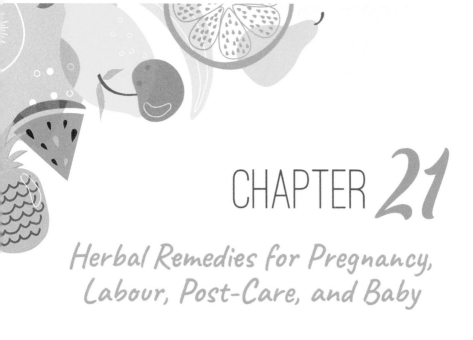

CHAPTER *21*

Herbal Remedies for Pregnancy, Labour, Post-Care, and Baby

Herbalism teaches that our bodies are incredible healing machines, hence allowing the body a chance to self-heal is incredibly important. Herbal remedies assist the body's natural healing abilities.

I am listing the mentioned options to be a talking point with your health practitioner. I have purposely left out how to make your own decoctions and tinctures due to the inherent dangers if not prepared properly. If you do need herbal products, I recommend seeing an Herbalist or a Naturopath and ask them to make a tincture that is suitable for your needs. Generally, a practitioner will make one specifically for you rather than just grab a ready-made one off of the shelf. If you're ever concerned, always seek medical advice.

Personally, I'm not a huge fan of mainstream homeopathic products because many of them are far too diluted to be considered therapeutic, but many herbs must be diluted to be considered safe. With homeopathic alternatives, many baby care products are far better than the conventional substitutes because they don't contain a lot of the nasties. If available to you, always purchase your homeopathic products from a homeopath, or from your local health store, and ask for assistance. Remember that essential oils are for external use only, and they must be added to a carrier oil, and/or diluted in water.

Herbs for Pregnancy (do not over consume)

- Ginger Tea. Anti-inflammatory, soothes the belly, and helps strengthen the immune system. Grate a small cube of fresh, peeled ginger and steep in hot water for five to ten minutes. Add cold water before drinking, if necessary. Drink one cup per day, or every second day, as needed.
- Dates. Eating six dates every day, from week thirty-seven of pregnancy, has been proven to help 'cervical ripening' for a shorter and smoother labour. I have personally tried this and found that it helped immensely. Recent studies can be found at www.nutritionfacts.org
- Pineapple. Fresh pineapple is said to help 'cervical ripening' due to the enzyme, bromelain. Do not eat large amounts during your pregnancy, but you can eat larger amounts closer to your due date.
- Rosehip Tea. Anti-inflammatory and full of phytonutrients, look for rosehip tea that isn't blended with other herbs. Best to drink after the first trimester.
- Rosehip Oil. Perfect for applying to the growing belly, rosehip oil is high in vitamin A, C, and E, and encourages elasticity to help alleviate stretch marks. Look for 100% organic rosehip oil that uses the whole fruit (many just use the seeds). Whole oils will generally be labelled 'Rosa Canina Fruit Oil' or will not mention anything about being the oil from the seed. It will also have a slightly red tinge, while refined and 'seed oil' will have a yellow tinge. Rosehip oil made in Southern Africa is renowned for using the whole fruit. Rosehip oil is a carrier oil (not an essential oil, so it doesn't have to be diluted), but to help it go further, you can mix a few drops with coconut oil or olive oil when applying to the belly. Apply small amounts up to twice per day.
- Echinacea. While it isn't recommended to take Echinacea tablets in large doses during pregnancy without seeking professional advice first, I keep 500mg Echinacea capsules on hand in case of viruses, bacterial infections, or severe flus. Echinacea has antiviral, antifungal, and antibacterial

properties and helps boost the immune system to fight illness naturally. In my experience, Echinacea works better for a cold or flu than antibiotics because of its antiviral properties. When I used Echinacea during pregnancy, I took two to three tablets of the powdered wholefood form, per day.

- Lemon tea (lemon wedges steeped in hot water) helps to alkalize the body, kick start and aid digestion, and also helps to relieve gas.

- While this isn't an herbal remedy, listening to Binaural Beats during pregnancy, and particularly during labour, helps in many different ways. Many people use Binaural Beats to de-stress, to help lose emotional baggage, to help raise their vibrations, and for meditation. During labour, Binaural Beats can help mama go into a light meditative state to help deal with labour pains. There are many free sources of Binaural Beats online.

Herbs for and After Labour

- Raspberry leaf (tea or tincture) is one of the best uterine tonic herbs to prepare uterine muscles for efficient labour. Its astringent action slows bleeding and helps to expel the placenta. Have the tea on hand to drink during labour.

- Rescue Remedy, a Bach flower remedy, is perfect if stress arises during labour.

- Lavender essential oil is calming and soothing. Mix one drop of lavender oil to every 10ml of carrier oil. Or dilute about five to ten drops of lavender in two cups of water (500ml). Do not apply undiluted oil directly to the skin. Some women find comfort in having the lavender water sprayed/misted on them during labour. Using lavender oil in an oil burner, or oil diffuser may help as well. Note: *directly applying lavender oil and lavender oil products to the skin has been linked to abnormal breast growth in men and children.*

- St. John's Wort Oil can be rubbed on the perineum at the time of delivery to help reduce tearing. Applying this oil after birth will also help heal any tearing as well. It has a soothing action and reduces burning and swelling. Many oils are already mixed, but you will have to mix it in a carrier oil if not. Follow the instructions on the back.

- If you are using a birthing bath, small amounts of magnesium salts can help contraction pain, the same way magnesium helps joint and muscle pain, if added to the water. These salts help relax and soothe the muscles and will help cleanse and heal the vagina once baby is born. There is conflicting information about magnesium stopping contractions and helping contraction pain. OB/GYN's used to prescribe magnesium IV shots and oral magnesium for women who went into early labour to stop contractions. However, bear in mind that an IV shot is far more intense and concentrated than adding magnesium to the water. Magnesium is also a natural blood thinner so adding smaller amounts as if you're swimming in the ocean, is key. If you naturally have thin blood, please do not opt for this method. Otherwise, if this is something you wish to consider, discuss this with your practitioner first.

Aftercare

- A magnesium salt sitz bath after delivery will help clean and heal you, especially if you've torn. These salts will also help reduce swelling. If you can, take a sitz bath at least once every day. This will speed up the healing process.
- Comfrey can also be added to the sitz bath and helps heal any tears and tenderness, and helps prevent infection. Comfrey tea can also be applied to the breast for breast infections.
- Chamomile tea helps soothe pain after labour and promotes sleep.
- Coconut Oil is perfect to wash the vagina with after labour. It's antibacterial properties help to keep infections at bay,

while also soothing the sting and swelling associated with a vaginal birth. It isn't recommended to use soap. Shower at least twice per day.

- **Arnica spray** is a natural pain reliever and can be used on the perineum after birth. Use with care.

Baby

It isn't recommended to give newborn babies herbs, especially in therapeutic doses. Babies should only be given breast milk, or non-toxic formula, until four to six months of age. Although many parents do use smaller doses of herbs to help with illnesses and infections, always seek professional advice. There may come a time when baby is sick, and you may not want to give baby standard medication; always ask your practitioner for advice before administering anything outside of baby's usual food, especially before baby is six-months-old. I have added a list of herbal remedies that mamas have successfully used to treat baby.

If breastfeeding, mama can take a half dose of the herbal remedy, or drink the herbal tea, and the benefits will flow to baby through mama's breast milk. Always use with care and ask your health practitioner for advice first.

- **Echinacea** has been known to help babies fight off bacterial and viral infections, something that antibiotic drugs cannot do. If baby has an infection or a fever, and if you do not want to administer antibiotic drugs, speak to your practitioner about safely administering Echinacea.
- **Coconut oil** can be gently massaged on to baby's feet to help calm and relax him. It is also my preferred baby soap and shampoo. When using coconut oil as a soap, there is no need to use a powder under baby's neck and armpits. Coconut oil also helps treat mild cradle cap. Wash babies scalp with the oil and rinse, once per week. The oil will make baby's hair greasy, just wash it out with water over the

next few days. Coconut oil also helps teething rash, minor irritations, and dry skin.

- **Chamomile** helps soothe teething pains, and can also be used to help colic, fever and stomach aches. Many homeopathic teething gels also contain chamomile (if opting to use homeopathic teething products make sure they **do not** contain **belladonna**, or that the company is transparent about heavily diluting belladonna in their products. For example, heavily diluted is one-hundred-fold, thirty times over, rather than ten-fold, three times over). Drinking chamomile tea helps relieve reflux, wind pain, and digestive discomfort in baby through mama's breast milk. Drink two to four cups when needed.

- **Catnip** is a relatively mild herb that can be used to help ease colds, flu and fevers.

- **Elderberry syrup and tea** helps boost the immune system and helps fight cold and flu symptoms. It acts as an anti-inflammatory which reduces swelling in the mucous membranes to help relieve congestion. It is recommended to use elderberry syrup for children ages one and up, unless prescribed by a reputable practitioner. If breastfeeding, drink the tea and its mild effects will flow through to baby. I make elderberry tea by steeping the dried berries in boiled filtered water for about ten minutes. Strain and pour the water into a mug, add sweetener if desired, and serve.

- **Vitamin C** helps boost the immune system and is a natural antihistamine. To help relieve mild allergies in baby, such as heat rash, add a scoop of food-made vitamin C powder to a glass of water or coconut water and drink. Drink two to three glasses per day, until baby's symptoms improve. Use this method if baby catches a cold too. The affects will flow through to baby in mama's breast milk.

- **Mullein leaf** is well-known for its healing affects on the respiratory system, and has been used to treat chronic coughs, bronchitis, whooping cough, asthma, sinusitis, congestion and hayfever. It is also a powerful anti-inflammatory. Mama should take mullein capsules if breastfeeding, or mix mullein leaf powder into baby's smoothie, juice or food. Please speak to your practitioner about dosage as that will depend on baby's weight and age.

- Sea moss has also been used to help heal the respiratory system. It is also full of essential nutrients that can be difficult to gain in other food. If breastfeeding, add sea moss powder to your smoothie. Otherwise, mix the powder into baby's smoothie, juice or food. Please speak to your practitioner about dosage as that will depend on baby's weight and age.

- Ginger root is a natural anti-inflammatory that can be rubbed on baby's gums to help soothe teething pains. Slice and peel a piece of fresh ginger and rub on baby's gums.

- Liquorice root (not the edible, candy kind) can be chewed on and naturally numbs the gums while baby chews it. Liquorice root looks like a small stick, and baby will need to be supervised when chewing this.

- Breast milk is a powerhouse food and it also contains healing properties. Many mamas successfully use their own breast milk to treat baby's rashes, and minor cuts and grazes.

- Amber necklaces are designed for older babies and are to be worn but not chewed on. Baby's body heat releases the succinic acid contained in the stones, which is a natural pain reliever and inflammation reducer. I absolutely swear by these necklaces. Amber has been used for centuries to provide relief to teething babies. There are different qualities of necklaces and a lot of fake amber necklaces on the market. If you do opt for this method, choose a necklace that has individual knots between each bead. This is a safety precaution in case the chain breaks, so there is only one loose bead rather than an entire necklace. Take the necklace off baby when he or she is not in your sight and when sleeping.

Mastitis

Echinacea is an excellent antibiotic herb that will help reduce mastitis. Echinacea purifies the blood, destroys viruses, and prevents the growth of bacteria. It helps build the immune system and fights infection, both bacterial and viral. Take at low or recommended doses during breastfeeding.

Candida/Yeast Overgrowth/Group B strep (GBS) positive* related issues

- **Raw coconut oil** has powerful antifungal and antibacterial properties and is safe to take while breastfeeding. Take one to two tablespoons orally, daily. If you have tested positive for GBS, use coconut oil as a vaginal wash. GBS must be dealt with both externally and internally via the digestive system.
- **Cinnamon** is a powerful antifungal and antibacterial. It can be added to many foods but can also be taken in oil form (post-pregnancy only) or as a tea.
- **Turmeric** is a powerful antifungal and antibacterial and can be added to many foods.
- **Echinacea** will kill candida-overgrowth in the gut, however, it is important to wait until after baby is born and when you're no longer breastfeeding to use Echinacea for this purpose, due to having to take in higher amounts.
- **Chlorella** helps clear up candida in the gut and helps destroy the GBS bacteria.
- **Raw garlic** also kills the GBS bacteria during pregnancy. If your stomach can handle it, crush one to two cloves and leave them to sit in a small glass of water for ten minutes, before drinking. You do not have to eat the garlic cloves.
- **Probiotics** help fight off candida and GBS. Take probiotics internally and vaginally.
- If you have tested positive to GBS, increase the amount of **vitamin C**-rich foods in your diet and even take a food-made supplement if required. Vitamin C will help your immune system fight off the unwanted bacteria.

* GBS and Candida are very much linked. Candida has been shown to be an independent risk factor for vaginal colonization by GBS. If you have or had a candida infection or overgrowth, then you will typically test positive for GBS. The current recommended treatment for GBS is administering intravenous penicillin into mama, when mama goes into labour, and it is re-administered every four hours until baby is born. The penicillin crosses the placenta into the umbilical cord and into baby.

While there are benefits to this method and protecting baby from the GBS bacteria upon birth, administering antibiotics to any baby also come with its own health risks. This includes destroying baby's microbiome, which is fundamental to baby's maturing immune system, and is dependent on many of the bacteria present in mama's vagina; however, the penicillin destroys the bad bacteria, as well as the good bacteria in mama's vagina. Some health care professionals are also concerned about the use of penicillin at birth developing into 'antibiotic resistance,' which leaves baby more susceptible to superbugs, as well as severe food allergies.

Many mamas have reported that their babies developed severe food allergies after being in labour, and on IV penicillin, for twelve+ hours. This means that they were given numerous doses of penicillin, and so were their babies. Breastfeeding has been shown to help restore some of baby's microbiome, but no studies have been conducted to show the long-term effects. If you have tested positive to the GBS bacteria and you do not want to administer IV penicillin, know that there are natural ways to kill the bacteria.

Many mamas that have tested positive to GBS have also successfully given birth without passing it on to their babies. If mama has treated GBS naturally, the midwives will be aware of this and will usually monitor baby after birth and check his temperature to make sure that he hasn't developed an infection. There is a very small chance that baby will pick up the bacteria, but if baby does, it can be serious. If baby does develop an infection, he will be immediately started on antibiotics. Please discuss naturally treating GBS with your health care professional. If you're ever in doubt, please treat the bacteria as suggested by the hospital.

Herbs to Help Breast milk Production (teas not oils)

- Chasteberry (Vitex agnus-castus)
- Fennel (only seeds and fruit, avoid fennel oil)
- Alfalfa tea (can be taken about six weeks before birth - do not overconsume or consume if you suffer from a hormone-related cancer, or autoimmune disease)
- Red raspberry leaf
- Blessed thistle (will increase milk supply)
- Marshmallow (will make milk richer with a higher fat content)

Foods, such as potatoes, sweet potatoes, brown rice, oatmeal, and green papaya can help breast milk production. Plenty of water and rest is also recommended, as fatigue can affect milk supply. There is also a mental aspect to breastfeeding; the hormone, *prolactin*, is released from the pituitary gland in the brain and is the signal which triggers breast milk production during feeding. You may also notice that your breasts begin to leak when you simply think about baby or when you hear baby cry. So, from a mental aspect, keep your spirits high and keep your thoughts about breastfeeding, positive.

Herbs to Avoid During Breastfeeding

- Although fenugreek is a very common breastfeeding aid, fenugreek contains coumarin (a vitamin K antagonist), and can upset baby's digestion and cause flatulence. It also contains blood-thinning properties which can be passed on to baby.
- Parsley, sage, peppermint, and spearmint are linked to drying up milk supply. Even menthol cough drops and peppermint candies have been known to decrease milk supply.
- All herbs in Chapter 15 should be avoided and only administered if prescribed by a reputable clinical herbalist.

Newborns typically have an immature digestive system, which means that many different foods can upset their stomachs, particularly certain proteins and highly acidic foods. In food, I advise to use spices in much smaller doses, particularly if baby is showing signs of reflux, and only stick with milder medicinal herbs, such as chamomile, echinacea and elderberry tea while breastfeeding. Small amounts of culinary herbs in cooking is okay, but always gauge baby's reaction to all food that you eat. If baby shows signs of an allergy, food intolerance, fussiness, painful gas, or reflux, you will need to reassess what you eat. Please keep in mind that ear infections are a typical sign of a food allergy.

Common plant-based trigger foods are peanuts, nuts, wheat/gluten, refined sugar, citrus fruits, acidic foods, soy, tomatoes, cruciferous vegetables, caffeine, chocolate, garlic, onion, spicy/hot foods, and mint. If baby has symptoms, keep a food diary and eliminate these specific foods from your diet, and reintroduce them later on. Common allergy foods should be eaten during pregnancy and while breastfeeding, so baby is less likely to develop a food allergy when it's time for solids, unless of course, they cause reflux or discomfort. Be mindful that it can take four to six weeks for all of the proteins to leave yours and baby's body.

While reflux isn't usually food related, if baby is showing signs of reflux, it could be because of mama's forceful let-down and oversupply. If so, let baby suckle until you feel your let-down and then let your milk go into a towel until the fast and forceful milk stops. It may help to massage the breast while doing so to help clear out any blockages. While feeding, turn baby's head to the side rather than have baby facing up. This will stop the milk from going straight down baby's throat, and any excess milk will drip straight out of baby's mouth. It will also help to feed baby at an angle, and sleep baby at an angle as well. Because baby's digestive system is immature, baby's stomach can't handle having the milk go down his throat too fast, which typically results in vomiting.

Lastly, always make sure to burp baby, as trapped wind and gas are often reasons why baby is unsettled, shows fussiness during feeding, has mild reflux, and arches his back while crying.

CANDY MARX, MH, HHP

Nursing Mother's Tea

1 part Raspberry leaves
1 part Blessed thistle
1 part Marshmallow root

Make a cold infusion by soaking two tablespoons of the above herbs in one litre of distilled or filtered water. Steep overnight. Drink three cups daily, or as needed.

Tip for breastfeeding mamas: weaning baby gradually, rather than quickly, gives the breast tissue time to restore properly which in turn helps to maintain mama's pre-pregnancy breast shape. In other words, if you wean slowly, your breasts will less likely sag afterwards!

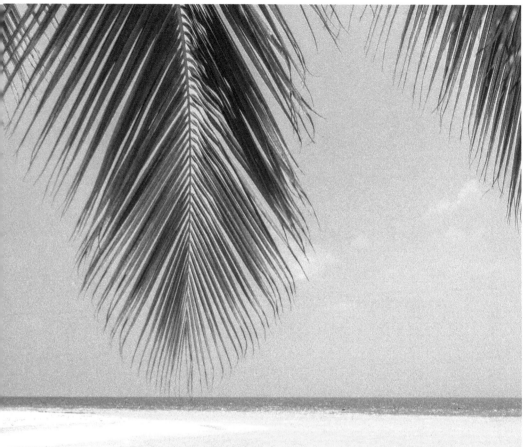

"Nature Itself Is The Best Physician."

- HIPPOCRATES

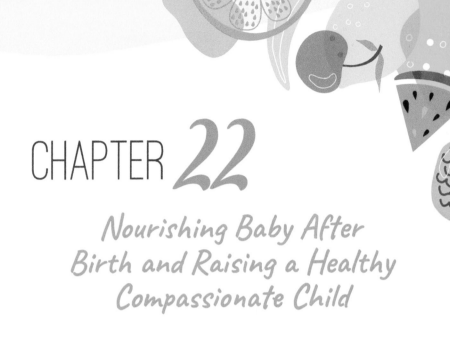

CHAPTER 22

Nourishing Baby After Birth and Raising a Healthy Compassionate Child

While it is crucial for mama to eat a wide range of wholefoods during pregnancy, it is equally important to keep this up during breastfeeding. This is how baby will get his nutrients. Be extra mindful of your vitamin K intake.

Colostrum is the first food that baby will eat. Every mama is different but mama will typically produce colostrum for the first one to five days after birth. The next stage is 'transitional milk' which typically lasts for ten to fourteen days. Transitional milk is a mixture of colostrum and breast milk, which will eventually be replaced by regular breast milk (foremilk and hindmilk). When the regular breast milk comes through it's important that baby gets plenty of hindmilk, which typically comes after the foremilk. Foremilk is watery-looking milk made up predominately of water and lactose. Hindmilk is rich-white milk and is where the good fats are. Hindmilk is how baby puts on weight. A good way to help baby drink the hindmilk is to feed from the same breast for two feeds in a row when starting to breastfeed. Too much of either milk can cause digestive discomfort so be sure that baby is getting a good balance of both.

Baby's stomach is about the size of a marble after birth, so it won't take much to fill it up. Many mamas worry that baby isn't eating enough, but if baby is feeding around eight times per day, and wetting about six nappies, then baby should be eating enough. Of course, always contact your health practitioner if you ever have any concerns.

For the first six months baby should only be fed breast milk. I understand that some women choose not to breastfeed or are unable to breastfeed. It is important to see your health practitioner to ensure you are nourishing baby properly. When using formula, always research the brand, as most formulas contain nasties and synthetic nutrients that baby will have trouble digesting.

The following table shows the composition of human colostrum, human breast milk, and cow's milk. Human milk is specifically designed for human growth, while, and this may come as a surprise to some, cow's milk is specifically designed for calf growth.

Compositions (g/L)	Human colostrum	Human breast milk	Cow's milk
Total protein	23	11	31
Immunoglobulins	19	0.1	1
Fat	30	45	38
Lactose	57	71	47
Calcium	0.5	0.3	1.4
Phosphorus	0.16	0.14	0.90
Sodium	0.50	0.15	0.41

Here is a typical feeding guide for baby. Use this as a guide only and seek professional advice when needed.

0 - 6 months: breastfed or non-toxic formula.

If baby isn't getting enough from milk alone, introduce solids before six months, but after four months. If you're unable to breastfeed but you can't or don't want to give baby formula, speak to your holistic practitioner about hemp milk, sea moss and coconut water/milk. See notes further on.

6 - 8 months: puréed fruit including vitamin K-containing fruits, high alkaline fruit such as raw banana, papaya, mango, watermelon, avocado, fresh coconut, hemp seeds (puréed with fruit), cooked/peeled apple, pear, mashed peas, filtered water, and breast milk (or non-toxic formula). Cooked and puréed mushrooms, as well as vegetables including pumpkin, sweet potato, carrot, silverbeet (swiss chard), kale, and dark leafy greens. Cruciferous vegetables must be cooked properly. Lesser amounts of mashed lentils (red lentils are easy to mash) that have been prepared properly. Baby will now need the iron from the legumes and dark leafy greens. Try plain purées at first to make sure baby doesn't have an intolerance. You can begin to introduce small amounts of culinary herbs to baby's meals, including ginger. When I introduce nuts, I let baby lick them first. You'll know when baby starts solids, he's usually keen to taste test everything, and allowing baby to lick them first will allow mama to see if baby reacts to it. If no reaction occurs, then I add small amounts of nut butter to baby's food. See note about common allergy foods further on.

* *While baby is still in the womb, he stores iron in his liver which will help him until four to six months after birth. Continuing with breast milk and adding vegetables paired with fruit or vitamin C vegetables will help baby's iron absorption and iron stores.*

8 - 12 months: puréed fruit, avocado, fresh coconut, vegetables, and dark leafy greens, mushrooms, and smoothies (add small amounts of hemp seeds). Soaked and puréed well-mashed lentils, chickpeas, and peas. Legumes can be tough on baby's digestion, so make sure to prepare them properly and stick with easier-to-digest legumes until baby gets older. Soaked, cooked, and mashed low-phytic-acid-containing wholegrains and pseudograins, such as teff and buckwheat (make a porridge), filtered water, and breast milk (or non-toxic formula). Baby will need the iron from the legumes and wholegrains.

Note: Berries can cause irritation that looks like nappy rash. If your baby reacts to these foods, reintroduce them to baby's diet after nine months. Remove them from baby's diet if he shows signs of allergy or intolerance and see your holistic practitioner.

12 months+: a wide variety of smoothies (with hemp seeds), puréed fruits and vegetables, smaller amounts of soaked legumes, wholegrains, pseudograins, nut butters, seeds/seed butters, small amounts of culinary herbs and spices, small amounts of sea moss, filtered water, and breast milk if still breastfeeding. Fruits, vegetables, breast milk, and/or water should be the primary staple in baby's diet, accompanied by hemp seeds, legumes and wholegrains that have been prepared properly.

Note: It is recommended to gradually introduce common allergy foods, such as nuts, peanuts, wheat, and soy into baby's diet from six months of age. Delaying common allergy foods may increase baby's risk of developing allergies. However, eating common allergy foods while pregnant and breastfeeding is a great place to start! This is so baby's body gets used to the proteins that may cause trouble later on. Always take care with common allergy foods and keep an eye on baby to watch for an allergic reaction, such as a rash, hives, itchy skin, itchy eyes, or a runny nose. Administer food-made vitamin C (mixed with water or in a smoothie) to act as a natural antihistamine, and if needed, add small amounts of probiotics to baby's next few meals to help heal his gut.

If baby develops diarrhea, vomiting, swelling of the lips or face, experiences weakness/fainting, or is having trouble breathing or swallowing call an ambulance (paramedic) immediately. If you have nut allergies or any food allergy in your family history, make sure to ask your practitioner to test baby for allergies first. If baby has eczema, hayfever, asthma, or any condition that is triggered by allergens, he may be more susceptible to food allergies.

Additional Note: There is a lot of conflicting information about when to start baby on solids. Some experts recommend starting solids around four months, other experts recommend starting at six months. However, baby must be physically able to hold his head upright, without support. Head control is important in swallowing and self-feeding. Baby must also have lost his tongue-thrust reflex, so he can swallow food. Also, before six months, baby's gut microbiome is still building and developing. Giving foods that are hard to digest, too early, will affect baby's gut health, which will affect baby's immunity. Wait until baby is ready for solids, physically, mentally and internally. You'll know when baby is mentally ready for solids! If baby appears to be hungrier and not satisfied with only breast milk before six months, it could be because baby's appetite is growing and he is not getting enough nutrients. If baby is physically ready, and many are ready before six months, slowly introduce easy-to-digest-foods such as puréed cooked apple, banana, avocado, sweet potato (mixed with plant-milk to help lessen the hard-to-swallow starchiness), cooked greens, and pumpkin, alongside breast milk. Babies prefer sweeter foods, so try and start with vegetables first, as vegetables won't taste that great after eating fruit.

Personally, Kaimana was physically ready for solids at around five months of age, and when he showed interest in my food I let him taste it. Sometimes he was interested in my food, but mostly, he wasn't. His appetite increased a lot from around four-months-old so I knew he'd try solid foods before six-months-old. He was still primarily drinking breast milk at around six months, and solid foods were just a top up. At around six-and-a-half-months-old, he was then mentally ready for solids and wanted to try everything. Every time we ate around him, he squealed at us because he wanted to eat it, well lick it, too!

Baby should typically get enough nutrients (including B12) from breast milk if mama is eating right, so if it's a possibility to breastfeed, do so for as long as you can. I do believe that small amounts of cacao and chocolate are okay during pregnancy, but try and limit your intake while breastfeeding, as the theobromine can end up in your milk. Some chocolate is okay but not in large amounts, as chocolate is a common cause of reflux and gas in babies. Caffeine levels peak in the body about one to two hours after consumption, but metabolite levels for theobromine peak later at about ten to fifteen hours. If you're still eating chocolate and drinking caffeinated beverages, please keep this in mind, and always keep an eye on baby's reaction to it. If baby seems distressed, gassy or stimulated, stop eating chocolate immediately.

Home-made hemp milk and coconut milk are super nutritious options to give baby. If you're not confident about getting enough nutrients into baby, you can also fortify these milks with small amounts of food-made nutritional supplements. Fresh coconut water has a similar profile to breast milk, because breast milk is made from mama's blood, and coconut water is similar to blood. So much that in WWII, coconut water was used in blood transfusions when treating wounded soldiers. In some countries, fresh coconut milk is used as a substitute for formula.

Hemp milk boasts a higher nutrient profile from good fats, easily digestible proteins which include all of the amino acids, and decent amounts of calcium, magnesium, potassium, iron, zinc, phosphorus, and folate. Sea moss is also full of bioavailable vitamins, minerals and Omega-3. Fresh coconut milk boasts a high nutrient profile including lauric acid which is a fatty acid in breast milk. However, it contains much less calcium, which is essential for a growing baby. Speak to your holistic health practitioner about hemp and sea moss milk, and coconut milk and blending these milks together. Quantities will differ for every single baby depending on current diet, age, weight, and other contributing factors.

Another important aspect is to keep baby's exposure to other people at a minimum in the first six to eight weeks, from anyone who doesn't live in your home. People carry viruses, germs, and bacteria and having everyone show up for a cuddle after baby is born, isn't the best thing for baby. Allow baby's immunity to develop and strengthen first. Make sure that anyone who wants to cuddle baby washes their hands first, and never let anyone with a cold, flu, or contagious disease handle baby or be in close proximity.

I highly recommend all parents take a first aid course. There are plenty of courses online, and in person. Just knowing the basics, such as clearing baby's throat, or performing CPR, gives you the tools if you're ever in an emergency situation.

When it comes to raising vegan children, it is much easier than most think, especially when you know the nutritional side. With my own children, especially Keilana who is at school now, kids' parties can be a nightmare when it comes to food. However, if we educate our little ones from an early age and explain precisely what 'typical party foods are,' then they generally don't mind not eating it. Every time Keilana has had a friend's birthday party, I either make or buy a raw treat for her to take, so she doesn't feel left out. When her close friends have a birthday party, their parents usually cater for Keilana in some way, which has been fantastic.

For school lunches, I pack three to four pieces of fruit, a buckwheat muffin of some sort (either sticky date, banana and chocolate chip, or raspberry and coconut), home-made popcorn, besan wraps, home-made trail mix (nut-free of course), and/or leftovers from dinner. There is a nut restriction at school, but it is still easy to pack healthy nut-free and gluten-free lunches.

The following recipes are all child friendly and are Keilana's favourite recipes! Just swap out ingredients that your child may not like.

We are raising the next generation of leaders and changemakers. It's essential that our children are compassionate, healthy, and well-loved!

I know there is a lot of information in this book and it may seem overwhelming if you're only just starting out on your vegan journey. Take it one step at a time and refer back to this book when you need to. If you're ever feeling overwhelmed, lost, or in doubt, or if you just need advice, please join Plantfed Mama's forum (www.plantfedmama.com/forum) and chat with other vegan mamas around the world, myself included.

I hope that after reading this book you're more confident in your decision to have a plant-based pregnancy and raise a compassionate, healthy, and conscious child. If done correctly, plant-based and vegan mamas and children will absolutely thrive!

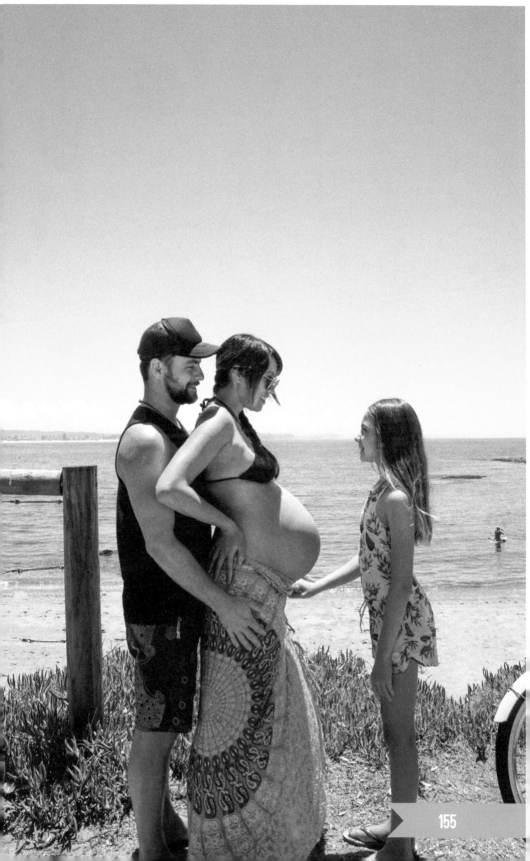

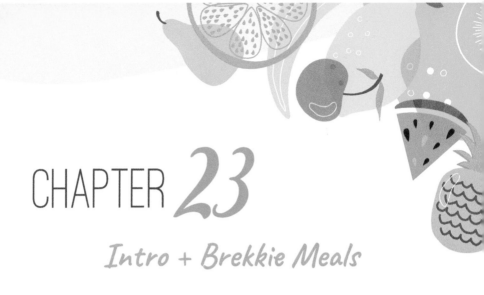

CHAPTER 23

Intro + Brekkie Meals

All of the following recipes are straight from my heart and have been created using wholefoods. The intention is to have loads of nutrients, including macros, micros, phytos and/or lifeforce, and of course, love, in every bite. I have paired these foods to increase nutrient absorption. As you will see, I don't use any gluten or refined sugars, and my recipes don't keep us in the kitchen for hours at a time, even though I like to make most foods from scratch.

Although cooked garlic and cumin were food aversions for me during my first and second trimesters, I have added garlic and cumin as optional in my recipes. If they aren't a food aversion for you, please feel free to add them.

I never make food that has zero nutritional properties. I can't make a flashy dessert just for the taste; there has to be some nutrients in any dish for me to make it. I also like to 'hero' the foods in my dishes, so you'll notice that many recipes don't contain a lot of ingredients.

If you're not a fan of cashews, you can substitute them with other soft nuts such as macadamias or Brazil nuts. And in some desserts, such as the cheezecakes, you can replace the cashews with fresh coconut.

I use raw mylk chocolate for ganache, and I prefer to make my own chocolate for desserts. If time is limited, just melt some raw organic chocolate instead. I use coconut butter for many of my desserts, instead of coconut oil, as coconut butter holds together better at room temperature. I also like that coconut butter uses the coconut meat, rather than just being an extracted oil, but you can use either.

Whenever my local farmer's market has overripe bananas, mangoes, or pineapple, I buy them in bulk. A handy tip is to peel, slice, and put them in a container in the freezer. Frozen bananas, mangoes, and pineapple are perfect for bowls, smoothies, and nicecream. I also keep organic frozen berries in the freezer as these always come in handy.

Use organic whenever possible, especially produce that is heavily sprayed such as berries, lettuces, green leafy vegetables, stone fruit, apples and pears, mangoes, cherries, kiwifruit, cucumbers, grapes, capsicum (bell peppers), tomatoes, celery, and even some potatoes. Grains are also heavily sprayed, so opt for an organic version if you can. Use activated nuts and seeds when possible, and for those worried about a spike in blood-sugar, opt for dates and date paste over other sweeteners.

I bake using a fan-forced oven, so all of my recipes are using fan-forced degrees. If you are using a conventional oven, you will have to add about 20C/68F on top of the noted temperature, or a conversion chart will help.

I add coconut yogurt or ginger to my recipes, especially in my brekkie recipes, to kick-start the digestive tract, assist gut-health and help the immune system. These recipes are meals that I eat and make for my family. I haven't added anything that I wouldn't eat myself.

From this lazy (practical) cook to you! xx

Bowls are my favourite way to eat fruit. They're super easy, tasty, full of nutrients and lifeforce, and versatile so you can change them to suit your tastes, and whatever is in your kitchen. I also love making food look pretty, because I love eating pretty food that's full of love, and bowls are the perfect chance to do so!

Mango Bowl

INGREDIENTS (SERVES 1)

2 bananas (fresh or frozen)
2 cups of frozen mango
1 small cube ginger (peeled)
1 - 2 Medjool dates (optional)
1/2 cup of filtered water
(can use coconut water)
Fresh fruit/hemp seeds/nuts/
activated buckwheat to top
Coconut yogurt

METHOD

Add bananas, mango, ginger, dates, and water to a blender and blitz until smooth and creamy. Pour mixture into a bowl and top with fresh fruit, hemp seeds, nuts, activated buckwheat, and coconut yogurt.

TIP

If you prefer a thick ice-creamy texture, use frozen bananas.

VARIATION

Swap the frozen mango with frozen strawberries for a deluxe strawberry bowl. Yum!

Berry Açaí Bowl

INGREDIENTS (SERVES 1)

2 bananas (fresh or frozen)
1 frozen açaí sachet
1 cup frozen berries
1 - 2 Medjool dates (optional)
1 small cube of ginger (peeled)
1/2 cup filtered water
Fresh fruit/hemp seeds/nuts/
activated buckwheat to top
Coconut yogurt (optional)

METHOD

Add bananas, açaí, berries, ginger, dates, and water to a blender and blitz until smooth and creamy. Pour mixture into a bowl and top with fresh fruit, hemp seeds, nuts, activated buckwheat, and coconut yogurt.

TIP

If you prefer a thick ice-creamy texture, use frozen bananas.

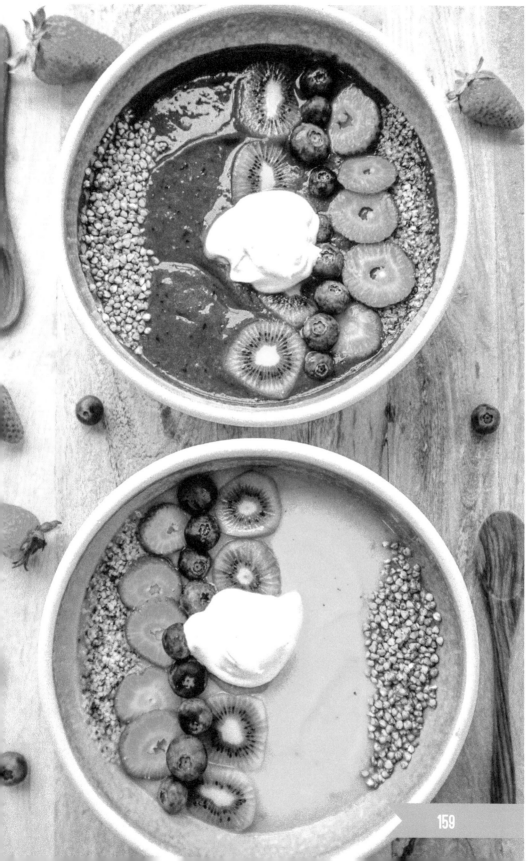

Pink Pitaya Bowl

INGREDIENTS (SERVES 1)

2 bananas (fresh or frozen)
1 fresh pink pitaya or
1 frozen sachet
1 small cube of ginger (peeled)
1 - 2 Medjool dates (optional)
1/2 cup filtered water
Fresh fruit/hemp seeds/nuts/
activated buckwheat to top
Coconut yogurt (optional)

METHOD

Add bananas, pitaya, ginger, dates, and water to a blender and blitz until smooth and creamy. Pour mixture into a bowl and top with fresh fruit, hemp seeds, nuts, activated buckwheat, and coconut yogurt.

TIP

If you prefer a thick ice-creamy texture, use frozen bananas.

Tropicana Bowl

INGREDIENTS (SERVES 2)

2 bananas (fresh or frozen)
1 - 2 açaí sachets
1 ripe mango (frozen)
2 cups ripe pineapple (frozen)
2 ripe passionfruit
1 - 2 Medjool dates (optional)
1/2 cup filtered water
Fresh fruit/hemp seeds/
nuts/granola to top
Coconut yogurt (optional)

METHOD

Add banana, açaí, mango, pineapple, dates, and water to a blender and blitz until smooth and creamy. Add passionfruit and hand mix with a spoon. Pour mixture into a bowl, and top with fresh fruit, hemp seeds, nuts, granola, and coconut yogurt.

TIP

If you prefer a thick ice-creamy texture, use frozen bananas.

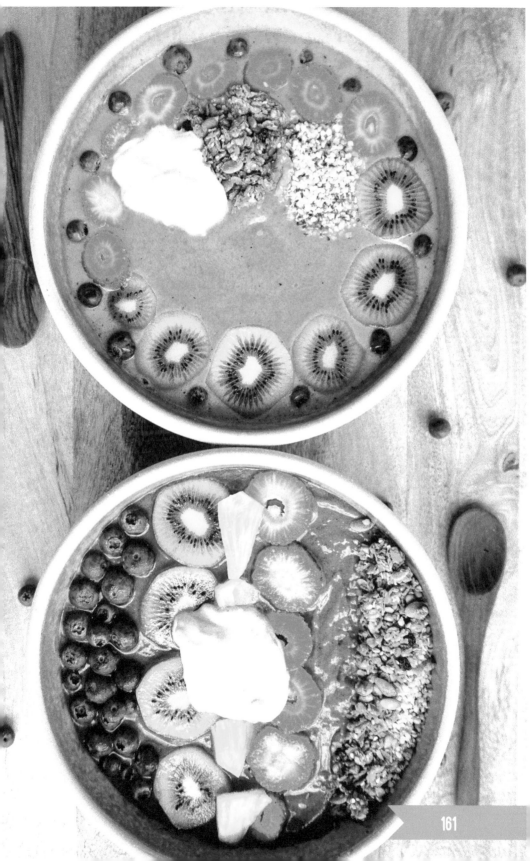

Mango Crepes
With Coconut Whipped Cream

I've remade my old pre-vegan favourite, mango pancakes, that are served at Yum Cha. Though this recipe tastes a lot better!

INGREDIENTS (MAKES 10 - 12 PANCAKES)

1 cup buckwheat flour
1 flax egg (optional)
1.5 cups plant-milk
1/4 cup coconut sugar (or preferred sweetener)
Tiny pinch pink Himalayan salt
2 ripe mangoes
Coconut Whipped Cream (see page 217)
Strawberry chia jam (optional, see page 195)

METHOD

Add dry ingredients to a bowl and stir. Make a well, add wet ingredients, and stir. The mixture should resemble a thick and sticky cake batter.

To a hot pan, add approximately 1/4 cup of pancake mixture and cook for 2 - 3 minutes on each side, or until the edges darken and bubbles appear on the surface.

Keep pancakes warm in the oven while cooking the rest of the batch. Prepare the coconut whipped cream.

Peel and slice the mangoes into long strips and layer inside each crepe then top with cream, then roll into cigars. Use a toothpick to hold in place if needed.

VARIATION

Use fresh strawberries instead of mango for strawberries and cream. Yum!

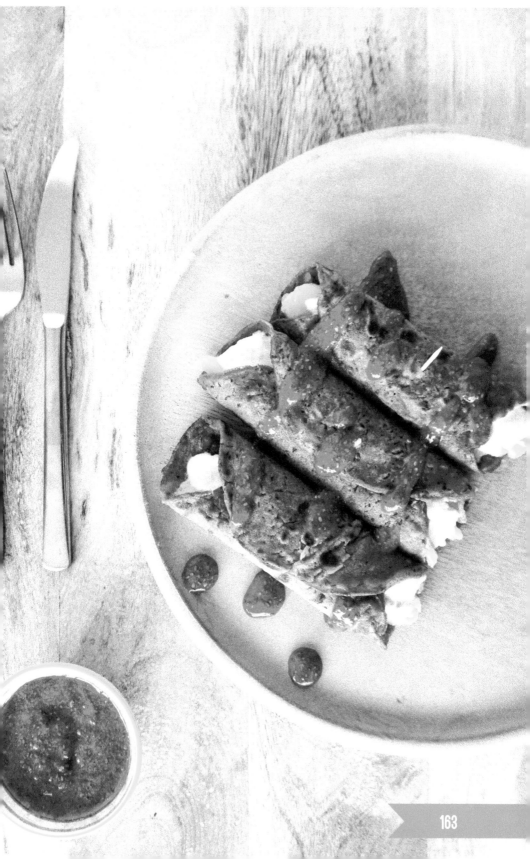

Tropical Fruit Platter

There's something special about eating from a platter and sharing it with loved ones. This simple platter of tropical fruit is full of lifeforce, enzymes, fiber, antiparasitic properties, and probiotics. Perfect for gut-health!

INGREDIENTS (SERVES 3 - 4)

2 bananas
1 - 2 ripe mangoes
1/2 ripe pineapple
3 - 4 ripe passionfruit
Handful strawberries
Handful blueberries
1 small papaya
Coconut yogurt to serve
Dash of fresh lime juice or orange juice

METHOD

Chop up the fruit and place on a large platter. Squeeze lime juice or orange juice over the papaya and serve with coconut yogurt.

TIP

Smaller papayas taste a lot better than their larger counterparts, so purchase smaller ones when you can.

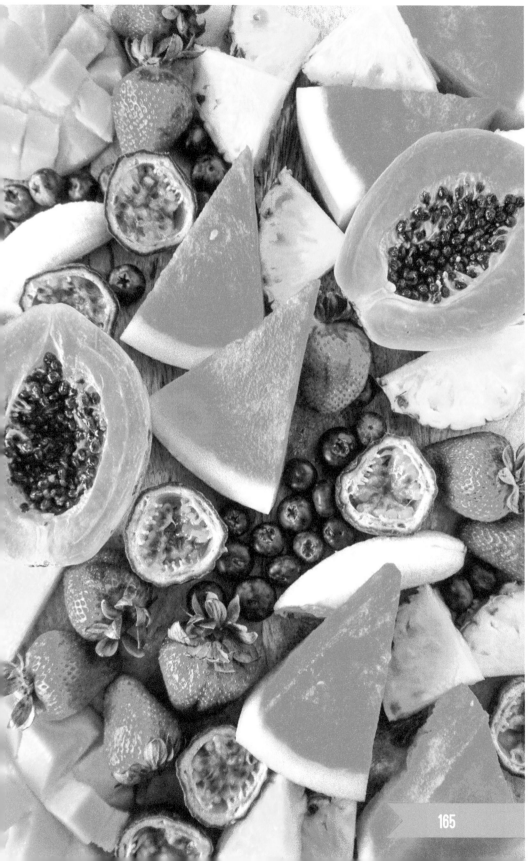

Buckwheat Porridge

Buckwheat porridge is very filling and a little goes a long way. This recipe serves two or one extra hungry person!

INGREDIENTS (SERVES 2)

1 cup raw or activated buckwheat groats (soaked overnight or at least 3 hours)
1 - 2 tbsp hemp seeds
3 - 4 Medjool dates (pitted)
3/4 cup - 1 cup plant-milk or filtered water
1/2 tsp ground cinnamon (optional)
1/2 tsp vanilla powder or extract
Fruit and nuts to top

METHOD

Rinse the buckwheat and add to a stick blender beaker or a medium bowl. Add hemp seeds, dates, milk, cinnamon, and vanilla. Blend until you get a thick porridge consistency. Adjust any ingredients if you need to. Pour buckwheat porridge into a bowl and top with fruit and nuts.

In cooler months, lightly heat in a saucepan before serving.

TIP

I find this recipe is easier to make using a stick blender rather than an actual blender.

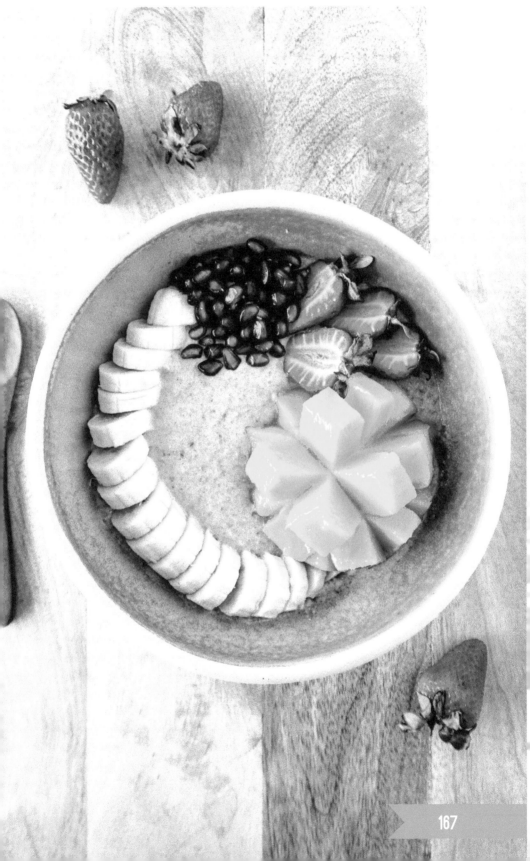

Home-Made Cereal

Aside from fruit, home-made cereal is one of my breakfast favourites. Wholefoods that naturally contain iron, calcium, and magnesium are better for you than fortified cereals that contain synthetic nutrients. Making cereal at home is super easy and you can add whatever you like! If you can't source dried mulberries, add chopped dates or raisins as they add a sweet chewy texture.

INGREDIENTS (SERVES 2)

1 cup dried white mulberries (make sure to take the sticks out)
Handful of activated or caramelized buckwheat groats
1/2 cup puffed amaranth
Handful almonds (chopped)
Handful cashews, pecans, macadamias or preferred nuts (chopped)
Handful shredded coconut
2 tbsp hemp seeds
2 bananas
2 Medjool dates (chopped) or 2 small handfuls of currants (optional)
Seasonal fresh fruit
Plant-milk to serve

METHOD

Divide ingredients between 2 bowls. Add mulberries, buckwheat, amaranth, nuts, coconut, and hemp seeds to a breakfast bowl and stir. Cut up the bananas, fruit and dates and place on top. Pour milk over the top.

VARIATIONS

Use whatever ingredients you have on hand and keep changing the recipe for something different.

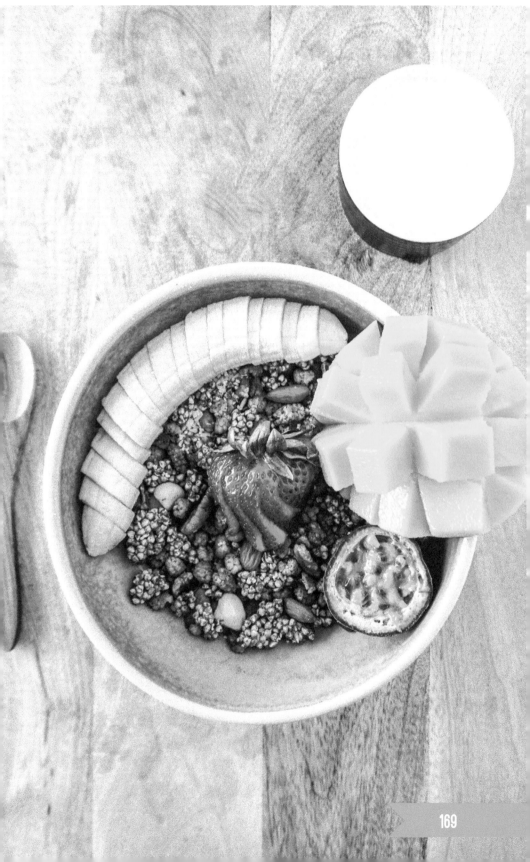

Veggie-Loaded Tofu Scramble

This recipe is a family favourite and is even loved by meat-eaters. Not only a nutritious and filling breakfast, it's also perfect for lunch and dinner as well.

INGREDIENTS (SERVES 4)

450g firm tofu
3/4 cup plant-milk
1 cup broccoli (chopped into small pieces)
1 cup cauliflower (chopped into small pieces)
1 cup green beans (sliced into quarters)
1 cup mushrooms (sliced)
Handful chopped shallots (scallions/green onion)
2 - 3 tsp ground turmeric
1/2 tsp paprika
2 cloves of garlic
2 - 3 tbsp tamari
Large pinch pink Himalayan salt
1 tsp Black Himalayan salt/Kala Namak for an egg flavour (optional)
Black cracked pepper
Preferred oil to cook with

METHOD

Add tofu to a large mixing bowl. Using the back of a fork, mash the tofu into small pieces. Add spices, garlic, and tamari and mix thoroughly. Add veggies and plant-milk, season with salt(s) and pepper and mix well.

Add mixture to a hot pan, stirring frequently. If mixture dries up, add more plant-milk. Cook for 10 - 15 minutes or until vegetables have softened and tofu is heated through.

Serve on gluten-free or sourdough toast, with a side salad, and sliced tomato.

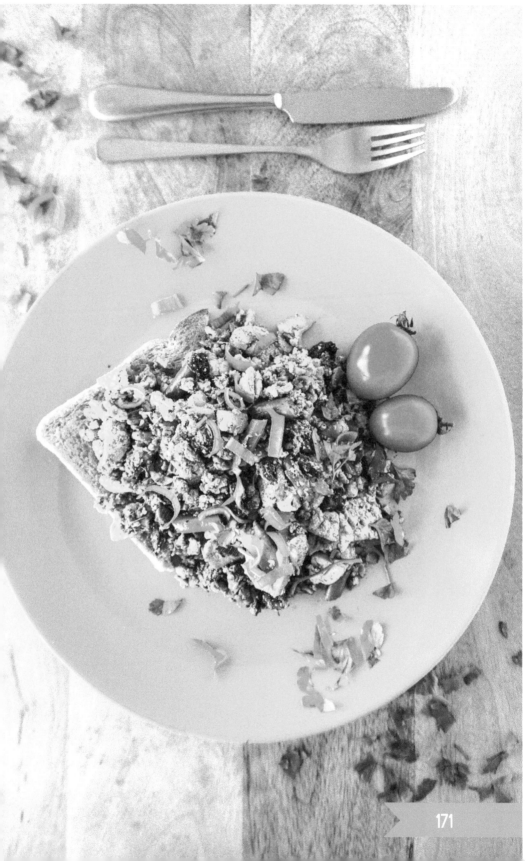

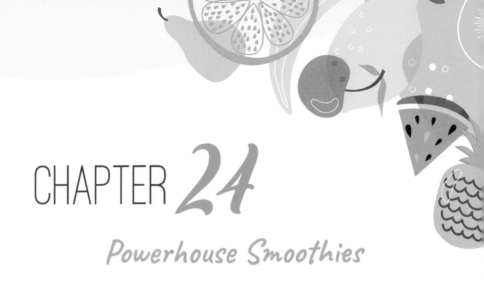

CHAPTER 24

Powerhouse Smoothies

Along with my beloved fruit, I like to add fresh beets to my smoothies. Beets are an excellent source of folate, amongst other nutrients, and are a powerful anti-inflammatory, detoxer, and blood purifier. When combined with fruit, you can't taste the beets at all. To me, smoothies taste better using frozen bananas, but in cooler weather, I use room temperature bananas. There is some misinformation about fiber being destroyed by blending it in smoothies, but this is not true. A professional, high-speed blender may break it down, but it doesn't destroy it. If anything, it is more likely to aid digestion.

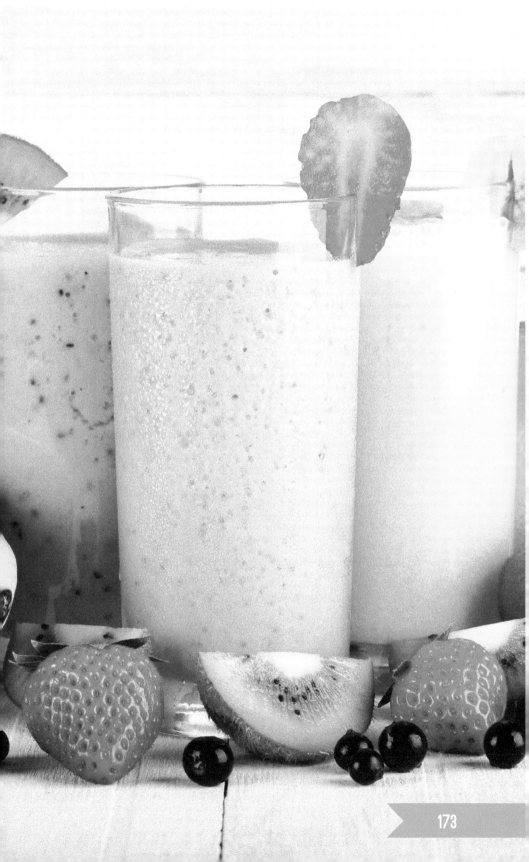

Pitaya Berry Beet

INGREDIENTS (SERVES 1)

1 - 2 bananas (fresh or frozen)
1/2 pink pitaya (or one frozen sachet)
1 cup blueberries or strawberries (fresh or frozen)
1 beet (cleaned and peeled, fresh or frozen)

1 small cube ginger (peeled)
Dollop coconut yogurt (optional)
2 tbsp hemp seeds
1.5 - 2 cups filtered water (or coconut water)

METHOD

Add all ingredients to a blender and blitz until smooth and creamy. If too thick, add more liquid and blend again.

Mango Passion

INGREDIENTS (SERVES 1)

1 - 2 bananas (fresh or frozen)
1 mango (fresh or frozen)
3 - 4 ripe passionfruit
2 tbsp hemp seeds

Dollop of coconut yogurt
1.5 - 2 cups filtered water (or coconut water)

METHOD

Add all ingredients except for the passionfruit to a blender and blitz until smooth and creamy. Pour into a glass and hand-mix the passionfruit into the smoothie.

TIP

If the passionfruit is sour, add a Medjool date or 2 before blending.

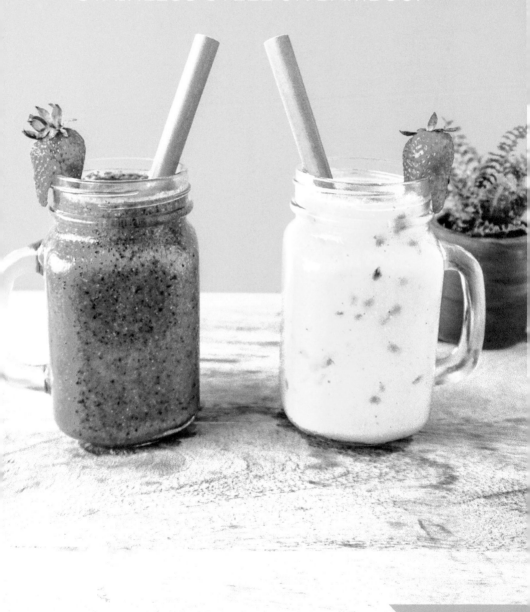

"DO YOU USE SINGLE-USE PLASTIC STRAWS? REPLACE THEM WITH STAINLESS STEEL OR BAMBOO!"

Beet Cleanser

This smoothie isn't for the faint-hearted. It's super cleansing and should be consumed at least twice per week.

INGREDIENTS (SERVES 1)

1 beet (cleaned and peeled)
The greens of one beet
(or 2 handfuls of baby spinach)
1 apple (cored)

1 small cube of ginger (peeled)
Half carrot (optional)
Juice of half a lemon
1.5 - 2 cups of filtered water
(or coconut water)

METHOD

Add all ingredients to a blender and blitz until smooth and creamy. Add more liquid if too thick.

TIP

Serve this smoothie in a jar with a lid. It will have fiber chunks and will separate. Shake and drink immediately.

Green Machine

INGREDIENTS (SERVE 1)

2 cups baby spinach (or preferred leafy greens)
1 banana (optional)
1/2 mango

1 cup fresh pineapple
1 tbsp hemp seeds
1.5 - 2 cups filtered water
(or coconut water)

METHOD

Add all ingredients to a blender and blitz until smooth and creamy. Add more liquid if needed.

TIP

Any time you add fresh greens to a smoothie, make an effort to chew the smoothie as greens need extra help from the enzymes in the saliva to help digestion.

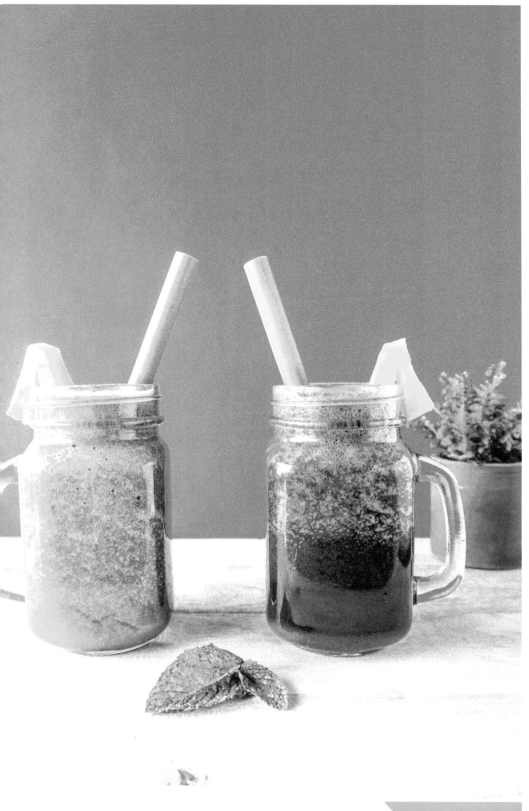

Salted Caramel

INGREDIENTS (SERVES 1)

2 bananas (frozen)
1 tbsp mesquite powder
1 - 2 Medjool dates (pitted)
1 heaped tsp almond butter
Small dollop coconut yogurt
Small pinch pink Himalayan salt
1.5 - 2 cups plant-milk

METHOD

Add all ingredients to a blender and blitz until smooth and creamy. Add more milk if needed and adjust to suit your tastes.

TIP

For an extra treat, rim the glass with Caramel Sauce (see page 260) before serving.

Creamy Coconut Rough

INGREDIENTS (SERVES 1)

2 bananas (frozen)
2 tsp cacao powder
1 - 2 Medjool dates (pitted)
1.5 - 2 cups plant-milk
Dollop coconut yogurt
1/2 cup shredded coconut
Pinch ground cinnamon
Sweetened cacao nibs (optional)

METHOD

Add all ingredients, except for the nibs, to a blender and blitz until smooth. Add nibs and roughly blend. Add more milk if needed and adjust to suit your tastes.

TIP

For an extra treat, rim the glass with chocolate sauce or Choctella (see page 196) before serving.

VARIATION

Replace the shredded coconut and coconut yogurt with 1 - 2 tbsp of smooth peanut butter or almond butter and 2 tbsp of hemp seeds or hemp protein powder, for a high protein Chunky Monkey Smoothie!

Pina Colada

This recipe is a family favourite. It's super simple and perfect for those hot days!

INGREDIENTS (SERVES 2 - 3)

1 large ripe pineapple
(fresh or frozen)
2 young/green coconuts
(or use 1 x 15 oz/400g BPA-
free can of coconut cream)
Additional water or coconut
water if needed.
Fresh mint (optional)

TIP

Taste the pineapple. If it isn't
quite ripe, add a dash of pure
maple syrup.

METHOD

Peel and chop the pineapple into small
chunks, removing the hard core from
the center. Add to a blender.

Open the coconuts and add the water
and the coconut meat to the blender,
or add the coconut cream instead, and
blend until smooth. Add mint if desired.
Add more liquid if you need to thin it out.

Serve with mint over ice in a garnished
glass.

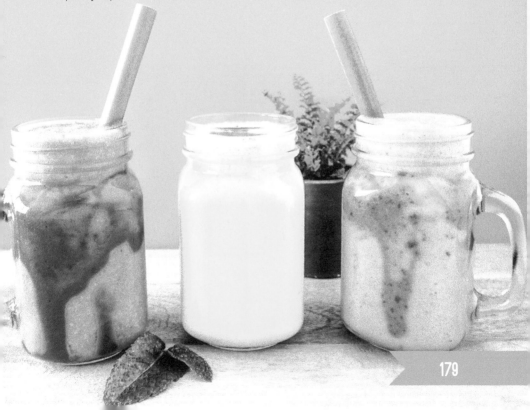

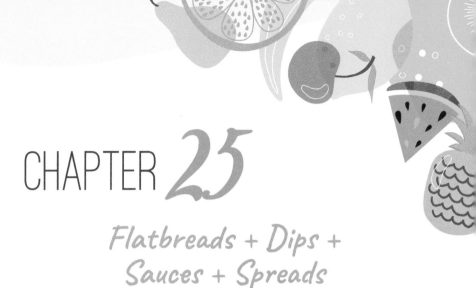

CHAPTER *25*

Flatbreads + Dips + Sauces + Spreads

Besan Wraps

These wraps are my absolute favourite, and they can double as savoury crepes. We've also used this recipe for pancakes too! They're super easy to make, taste great warm and cold, and are completely pliable. You can also make them ahead of time, stored in between paper towels, and they shouldn't fall apart.

INGREDIENTS (MAKES 5 - 6)

1 cup besan flour
1/2 cup tapioca flour/starch
Pinch pink Himalayan salt
Approximately 1 cup filtered water
Preferred oil to cook with

METHOD

Mix all dry ingredients together. Add water gradually. Set aside for 10 minutes. The consistency should resemble a pancake batter.

To a hot saucepan, add oil. Pour 1/4 cup of the mixture, cooking one at a time. Cook for 1 - 2 minutes on each side or until golden.

Serve alongside a curry or fill with legumes and salad and eat like a savoury crepe or tortilla.

TIP

I like to make these using 1/4 cups of batter, however make these wraps as small or large as you prefer.

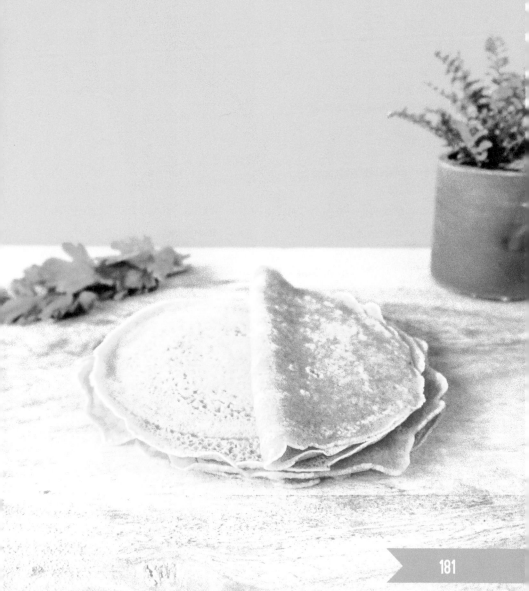

Besan Flatbread

I love Italian herbs and home-made flatbread, and this bread ticks both boxes! This recipe is super easy and tasty, just make sure not to overcook it as it will dry out.

INGREDIENTS (SERVES 2 - 3)

1 cup besan flour
3/4 cup filtered water
2 tsp olive oil
2 garlic cloves (crushed) or 2 tsp garlic flakes/powder
2 tsp dried Italian herb
Large pinch pink Himalayan salt

METHOD

Preheat oven to 180C/356F and line a flat baking tray with parchment paper.

Add flour and water to a bowl and mix till combined. Set aside for 10 minutes.

This step is crucial, so do not skip it as the besan needs time to thicken.

While the batter is thickening, mix the olive oil and garlic together. If using garlic powder, sprinkle on top with the herbs.

When the batter is ready, pour the batter onto the prepared tray. The consistency should be similar to pancake batter. Drizzle the garlic olive oil on to the batter, and sprinkle with herbs and salt.

Bake for about 12 - 15 minutes or until edges are golden brown.

Serve warm with fresh tomato and basil, soup or dips.

VARIATION

Replace the Italian herbs with fennel seeds for an Indian style flatbread and serve with a curry.

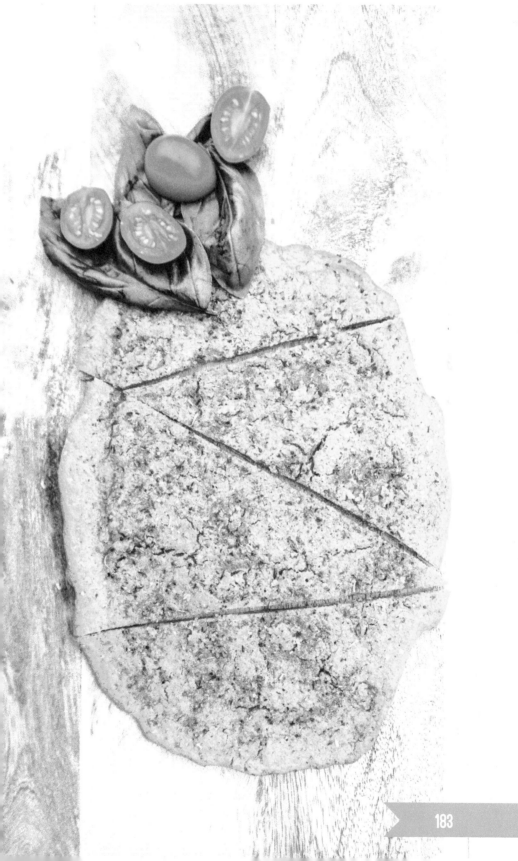

Home-Made Tortillas

Masa harina is corn that has been soaked in limewater before being ground into a meal. Soaking the corn first releases more nutrients and destroys the enzymes that are tough to digest. Masa harina is not the same as corn flour.

INGREDIENTS (MAKES 12 - 14)

2 cups masa harina
1 cup filtered water
Preferred oil to cook with

SERVE WITH

Tijuana Mexi Mix (see page 238)
Guacamole (see page 185)
Cashew Sour Cream (see page 216)

METHOD

Add masa harina to a bowl and add water gradually to form a dough. Roll dough into a ball, put in a sealed container and place in the fridge for 1 hour. Add a small amount of water if necessary. Note, some masa harina does not require being chilled first.

When the dough is ready hand roll into small balls. With a rolling pin, roll balls into tortillas. I find it easiest to roll the tortillas in between two pieces of parchment paper.

To a hot pan or skillet, add one tortilla at a time and cook for 1 - 2 minutes on each side, or until golden. Keep tortillas warm in the oven, wrapped in a damp tea towel so they don't dry out.

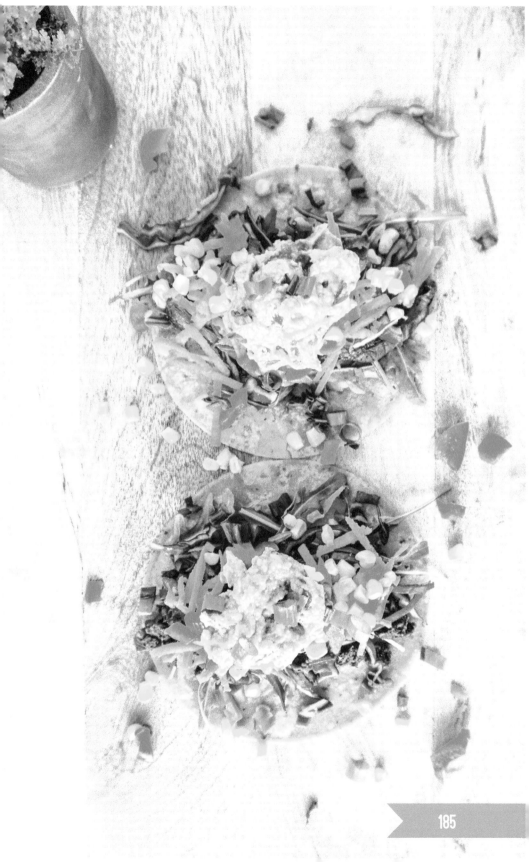

Sweet Potato Flat Bread/Wraps

INGREDIENTS (MAKES 2 LARGE WRAPS/ FLATBREADS OR 4 SMALL PITA SIZED BREADS)

1/2 - 3/4 cup mashed sweet potato
1 cup besan flour
1/2 cup tapioca or arrowroot flour
Pinch pink Himalayan salt

This is my absolute favourite flatbread. It's super easy to make and the dough can be made ahead of time and stored in an airtight container in the fridge.

METHOD

Preheat oven to 200C/ 392F.

Add half of a cup of sweet potato to a bowl and then add the rest of the ingredients. Mix until a dough forms. The dough should be moist but not sticky. Add more potato or flour if needed.

Split dough into 2 or 4 equal-sized balls and roll into flat discs, about 0.5cm thick, don't roll them too thin. Roll in between 2 pieces of parchment paper or on a floured surface.

Place on a large oven tray lined with parchment paper. If making 2 wraps, bake for 5 -7 minutes on one side. There is no need to flip the bread. If making 4 flat breads, bake for 3 - 5 minutes on one side. Keep an eye on them. The bread shouldn't become crispy. If it starts to become crispy, remove from oven. Keep in a clean damp towel until ready to use.

To serve, fill with lentil patties or loads of salad and Avocado Mayo (see page 192) or slice into fingers and serve with Hummus (see page 188) and Guacamole (see page 185).

VARIATIONS

After rolling out the dough, cut the dough into equal-sized discs and use as burger buns. The baking time will be about 2 - 3 minutes or so. This recipe can also be used as a pizza base and gnocchi! Or bake with Italian herbs, olive oil, garlic, and a pinch of pink Himalayan salt for an Italian-style flat bread.

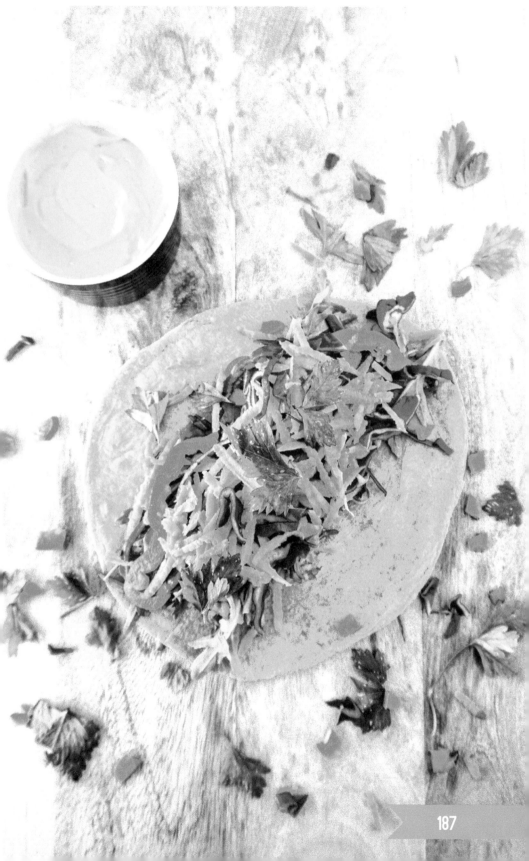

Hummus

Hummus is best made at home!

INGREDIENTS (MAKES APPROXIMATELY 250G)

2 cups chickpeas (soaked and cooked) or 1 x 15oz/400g BPA-free can
2 tbsp tahini (unhulled)
1/2 garlic clove (can use garlic powder)
2 - 3 tbsp lemon juice
1 tsp cumin
Pinch pink Himalayan
1/4 cup olive oil, plus extra to serve
Paprika to serve

METHOD

Add all ingredients to a food processor and blitz until smooth and creamy.
Add hummus to a bowl and top with a dash of olive oil and a pinch of paprika.
See recipe image on page 200.

Guacamole

This recipe is proof that simple recipes are best!

INGREDIENTS

2 large ripe avocados
2 tomatoes (chopped)
Handful of chopped shallots (scallions/green onions) or 1/2 Spanish onion (chopped)
Pinch cumin (optional)
Pinch pink Himalayan salt
Pinch black cracked pepper

METHOD

To a bowl, add avocado and mix until creamy. Add tomatoes, shallots, and seasoning and mix again.

Serve with potato wedges, nachos, tortillas (see page 185), Sun Bowls (see page 219), or Tijuana Sweet Potato Boats (see page 238)!

See recipe images on pages 185/239.

Easy Tomato Relish

I don't like using store-bought tomato sauce, and this easy relish is the perfect replacement. Make sure to use sugar rather than liquid sugars like maple syrup, otherwise the relish will be slightly watery and won't be as flavoursome.

INGREDIENTS (MAKES APPROXIMATELY 300G)

1 Spanish onion
1 large garlic clove (this relish needs garlic)
3 - 4 large ripe tomatoes (chopped)
2 tbsp coconut sugar
2 tbsp apple cider vinegar
Large pinch pink Himalayan salt
Preferred oil to cook with

METHOD

Sauté onion in a hot pan, and then add garlic. Add tomatoes, sugar, apple cider vinegar, and salt and stir again. Keep on heat until mixture has thickened which should take about 15 - 20 minutes.

Keep the texture as is or roughly blend with a stick blender. Store in an airtight container in the fridge for about a week.

Serve with veggie burgers.

TIP

Although the tomatoes don't need to be peeled, some prefer to peel the tomato skin off for relishes. To peel the tomatoes, cut a 'cross' on one end of the tomato and soak the tomatoes in boiled water for about 2 minutes. The skin will naturally begin to peel making the tomatoes easier to peel.

See recipe image on page 231.

Cashew Mustard Dip + Aioli

Home-made dips always trump store-bought dips, and this dip is full of flavour! I love pairing this with home-made wedges.

INGREDIENTS

1 cup cashews (soaked for at least 2 hours)
3 tbsp lemon juice
1 - 2 tbsp Dijon mustard
1/2 cup filtered water
Large pinch pink Himalayan salt

METHOD

Add all ingredients to a blender and blitz until smooth and creamy. Depending on the brand, Dijon mustard can be quite strong, so add gradually to taste.

Store in an airtight container for about 1 - 2 weeks.

VARIATIONS

For aioli, add 1 - 2 cloves of garlic and blend until smooth. Use garlic powder for a less intense flavour.

See recipe image on page 201.

Avocado Mayo

Just like home-made dips, home-made mayo also trumps store-bought mayo. This mayo is super simple, and you may be surprised by how much it actually tastes like mayo!

INGREDIENTS

1 large avocado
2 - 3 tbsp olive oil
2 tbsp fresh lemon juice
1 garlic clove (use garlic powder if you don't like raw garlic)
1/2 tsp Dijon mustard
Large pinch pink Himalayan salt
1/4 tsp paprika

METHOD

Add all ingredients to a blender and blitz until smooth and creamy. Store in an airtight container for about 1 week.

VARIATION

Replace the avocado with 1 cup of soaked cashews or macadamias for a nut mayo!

See recipe image on page 187.

Almond Satay Dipping Sauce

This sauce is super versatile. Use it as a dipping sauce or pour over your favourite plate of veggies.

INGREDIENTS

1/2 cup almond butter (can use tahini or peanut butter)
2 - 3 tbsp tamari
1 tbsp pure maple syrup or 2 - 3 Medjool dates
1/4 cup apple cider vinegar
2 - 3 tsp fresh lemon or lime juice
1 tbsp ginger (grated)
1 garlic clove
1/8 cup olive oil (can replace with water if preferred)
Approximately 1/8 - 1/4 cup filtered water (to reach desired consistency)

METHOD

Add all ingredients to a blender or food processor and blitz until smooth and creamy. Adjust to suit your tastes.

Serve with Thai Summer Rolls (see page 202) or Raw Pad Thai (see page 220).

See recipe image on page 203.

Dijon Maple Dressing

A fresh and zesty dressing that's perfect for salad!

INGREDIENTS

1 part Dijon mustard
1 part pure maple syrup
1 part fresh lemon juice
2 parts olive oil

METHOD

Mix all ingredients until smooth and creamy. Store in the fridge in an airtight container.

Serve over salad.

See recipe image on page 219.

Strawberry Chia Jam

When you see how easy it is to make jam, you'll never want to buy it again!

INGREDIENTS

2 punnets of strawberries (stalks removed, chopped)
2 tbsp pure maple syrup
1 - 2 tbsp lemon juice
1 - 2 tbsp chia seeds (or 1/8 tsp agar agar)

METHOD

For a raw jam, add strawberries, maple, and lemon juice to a blender or food processor, and blitz until smooth. Gradually stir in chia seeds and set aside to allow to thicken. Add more chia, if needed. Store in an airtight container in the fridge for up to 1 week.

For a longer lasting cooked jam, sauté strawberries in a saucepan, and add maple syrup and lemon juice. Use a potato masher to break up the strawberries. Add 2 tbsp of chia seeds and continue to cook until thick. Allow to cool.

If using agar agar, replace the chia seeds with agar and cook for 5 - 10 minutes until thickened. Agar agar must be cooked. Allow to cool. Store in an airtight container in the fridge for about 2 - 3 weeks.

See recipe image on page 162.

Choctella

A better and healthy version of an old childhood favourite that I eat by the spoonful!

INGREDIENTS (MAKES APPROXIMATELY 210G)

1 cup hazelnuts (raw or activated)
1/8 cup cacao powder
1/4 cup pure maple syrup
1/2 tsp vanilla extract
1/2 cup plant-milk
1 tbsp coconut butter or oil (melted)

METHOD

Preheat oven to 160C/320F. Spread hazelnuts on a baking tray lined with parchment paper and bake for 10 minutes, or until browned. Allow to cool slightly then rub the skins off.

Add hazelnuts to a food processor and blitz until a butter forms. Hazelnuts will turn to crumbs first but keep processing and a butter will form. If you do not have a food processor, crumb the nuts in a blender, and then pour the crumbs into a bowl and use a stick blender until a butter forms.

Add the rest of the ingredients and blitz until smooth and creamy. Adjust any ingredients if you need to. Store in an airtight jar in the fridge for up to 2 weeks.

This tastes amazing served over nicecream or used as a choc-hazelnut fondue. Yum!

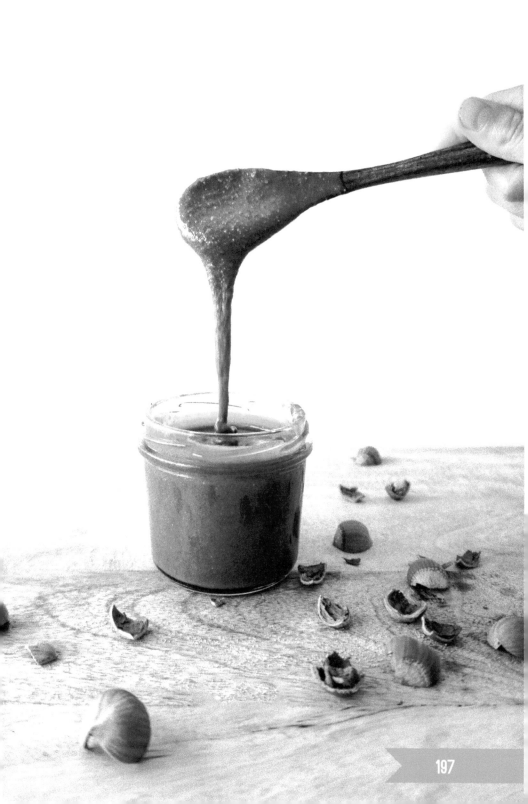

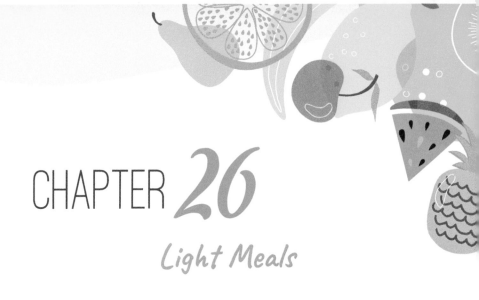

CHAPTER 26

Light Meals

Zucchini & Sweet Corn Fritters

I prefer to hero the corn in this dish, so I don't add too many ingredients or any spices, but you can add cumin or paprika for something different.

INGREDIENTS (SERVES 3 - 4)

2 zucchini (grated)
1 sweetcorn (kernels cut from cob)
1/2 cup chopped shallots (scallions/ green onions)
1 garlic clove
1 cup besan flour
Handful fresh parsley (optional)
Pinch pink Himalayan salt
Pinch black cracked pepper
Preferred oil to cook with

METHOD

Sauté the corn in a small saucepan and season. You can use raw corn, however, cooking the kernels first brings out the flavour. Add all other ingredients to a large bowl, mix well, and let the mixture sit for about 10 minutes. This step is crucial because the besan flour will soak up the moisture and create a batter. Then fold in the corn kernels.

To a hot pan, scoop out about 2 tbsp per fritter and add to a pan. Cook for 3 to 4 minutes on each side, or until golden brown and cooked in the center.

Serve with salad and Guacamole (see page 185) or Tomato Relish (see page 190).

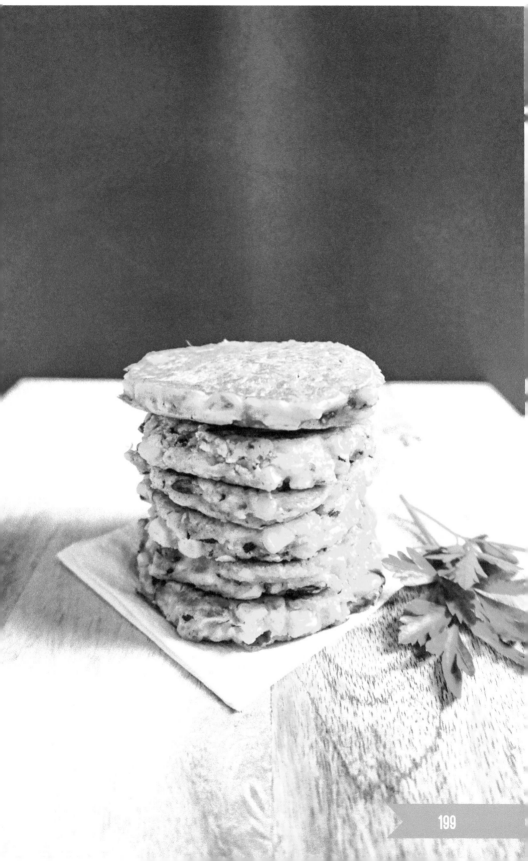

Paprika & Cinnamon Potato Wedges

This combo may shock a few of you, but it's a perfect combination of savoury with a hint of sweet!

INGREDIENTS (SERVES 3)

2 large sweet potato (orange sweet potato roasts best)
2 tsp smoked paprika
2 - 3 tsp ground cinnamon
1 - 2 tsp coconut sugar
Pink Himalayan salt
Dash of oil to cook with

METHOD

Preheat oven to 200°C/392°F. Line a large flat tray with parchment paper.

Wash potatoes and cut into wedges. Leave the skin on if you can. Add wedges to a bowl and top with the rest of the ingredients. Use your fingers to rub in the spices and coat the wedges thoroughly.

Bake for 30 - 35 minutes, making sure to turn the wedges every 10 minutes, to ensure the wedges do not become soggy. Allow to slightly cowol before serving.

Serve with a side salad, Hummus (see page 188), Cashew Mustard Dip (see page 191) or Guacamole (see page 185).

TIP

To make extra crispy wedges, add 1 tsp of instant polenta to the spice coating.

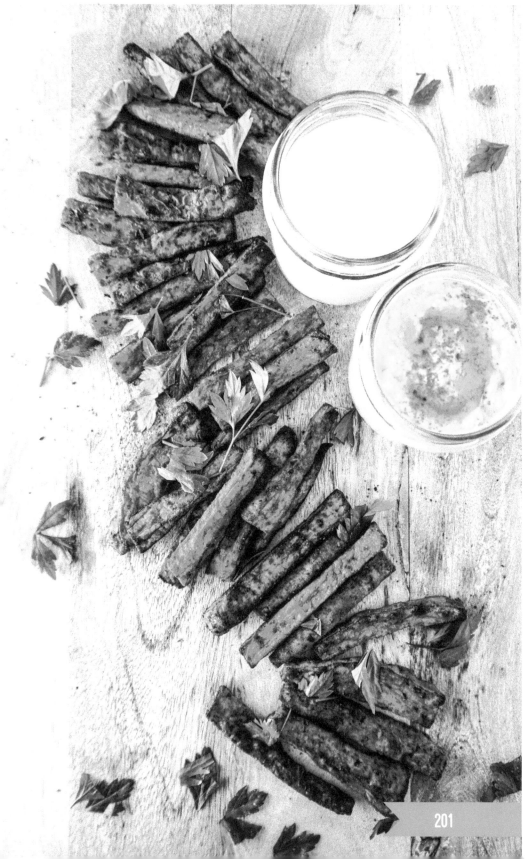

Thai Summer Rolls

I absolutely love these summer rolls. They're super easy to make, nutritious, and versatile. This recipe is a favourite among children and adults - a true crowd pleaser!

INGREDIENTS (MAKES 8 - 10 ROLLS)

450g firm tofu
Handful any salad greens
1 red capsicum (thinly sliced)
1 carrot (thinly sliced)
1 - 2 cups red cabbage (thinly sliced)
Handful fresh mint
Pink Himalayan salt
Black cracked pepper
Dried rice paper rolls
Almond Satay Dipping Sauce (see page 193)

METHOD

Preheat oven to 200C/392F. Slice tofu into 2cm baton strips and place on a baking tray lined with parchment paper. Season with salt and pepper, and coat with a splash of oil. Bake for 10 -15 minutes or until golden brown. Do not overcook as tofu will become dry.

Prepare the dipping sauce and vegetables.

Prepare the rice paper according to packet instructions. In the middle of the wrap, add greens, then tofu, then add the rest of the vegetables, ending with avocado.

Serve with Almond Satay Dipping Sauce (see page 193).

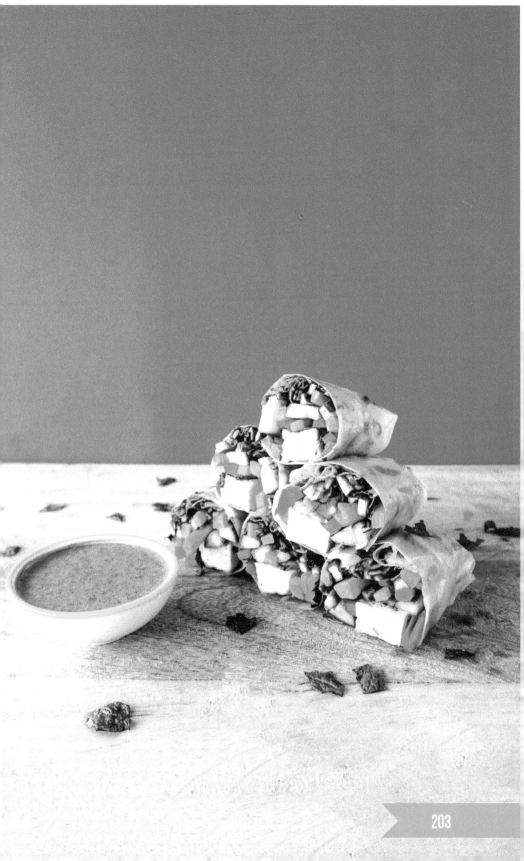

Curried Potato Cakes

These potato cakes are super simple and delicious. Add garden peas, corn, or whatever suitable vegetables you have in the kitchen.

INGREDIENTS (MAKES 8 - 10)

4 - 5 medium potatoes (peeled, cubed and cooked with salt, then drained)
1/2 cup besan flour
1 tbsp curry powder
1 - 2 tbsp plant-milk
1 tbsp date syrup or pure maple syrup (optional)
Handful of chopped shallots (scallions/green onions) or 1/2 Spanish onion (chopped)
Pinch pink Himalayan salt
Pinch black cracked pepper
Preferred oil to cook with

METHOD

Add potato, besan, curry, and seasoning to a large bowl. Mix with a fork, add plant-milk, and mix again. Fold in shallots or onion. The mixture should be sticky but should form into balls. If too wet, add more flour and adjust seasoning. If too dry, add more milk.

Roll into balls and flatten into patties. Add to a hot pan and cook for 3 - 5 minutes on each side, or until golden.

Serve with a huge side salad and Tomato Relish (see page 190) or Guacamole (see page 185).

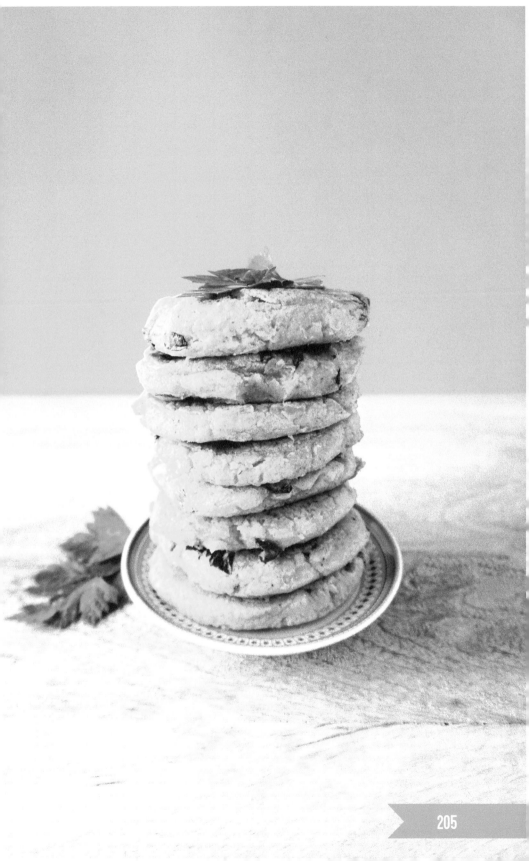

Raw Bolognese

I love this sauce. I make it with and without sun-dried tomatoes, so adding them are optional but they help thicken the sauce.

INGREDIENTS (SERVES 3 - 4)

6 large zucchinis (peeled and spiralized)
Approximately 8 large tomatoes
4 - 6 Medjool dates (pitted)
3/4 tsp - 1 tsp ground cumin
3/4 tsp sweet paprika
Pinch pink Himalayan salt
2 or 3 sun-dried tomatoes (optional)
Fresh basil and pine nuts, to serve

METHOD

Add all ingredients except for the zucchini, basil and pine nuts to a blender. Blend till thick and smooth. Adjust to suit your tastes.

Pour sauce over zoodles and mix thoroughly. Mix ripped basil through and serve in bowls. Top with toasted pine nuts and fresh basil. The fats from the nuts will help balance out the acidity and will also help nutrient absorption. If you have nut cheese, add the nut cheese to the top!

TIP

When working with zucchini noodles, the water content can make the sauce runny. If this is an issue, drain the zoodles in a strainer before adding the sauce. I usually place a cup underneath the strainer and push the noodles down, catching the water in the cup. Drink the nutrient-dense water instead of tipping it down the sink.

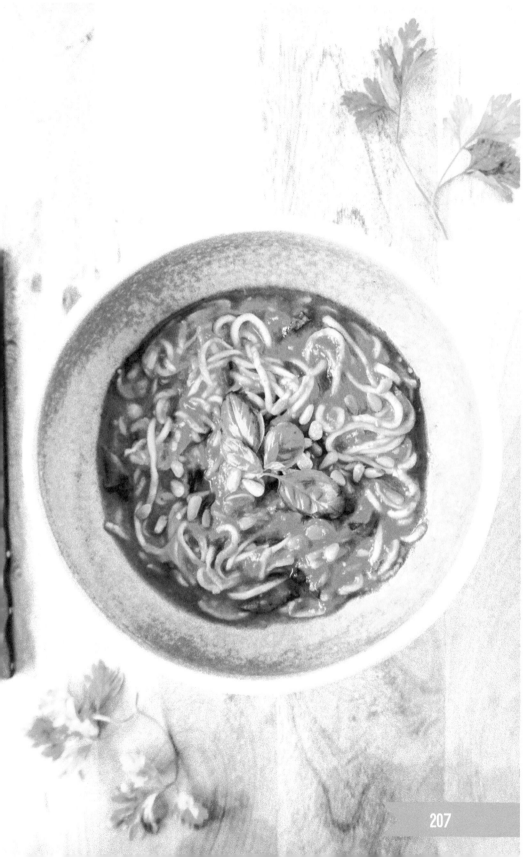

Watermelon Mint Magic

This is a delicious recipe and adding mangoes makes it even better.

INGREDIENTS (SERVES 2 - 4)

1/2 small watermelon
Fresh orange or lime juice
Handful of fresh mint
Coconut yogurt to serve

METHOD

Cut watermelon in half, lengthways. Carefully scoop the watermelon on to a chopping board, keeping the 'rind bowl' intact. Cut the watermelon into cubes or fruit balls. Add watermelon back into rind bowls, squeeze fresh orange or lime juice over the top, then add the mint and lightly mix with your hands. Top with coconut yogurt before serving.

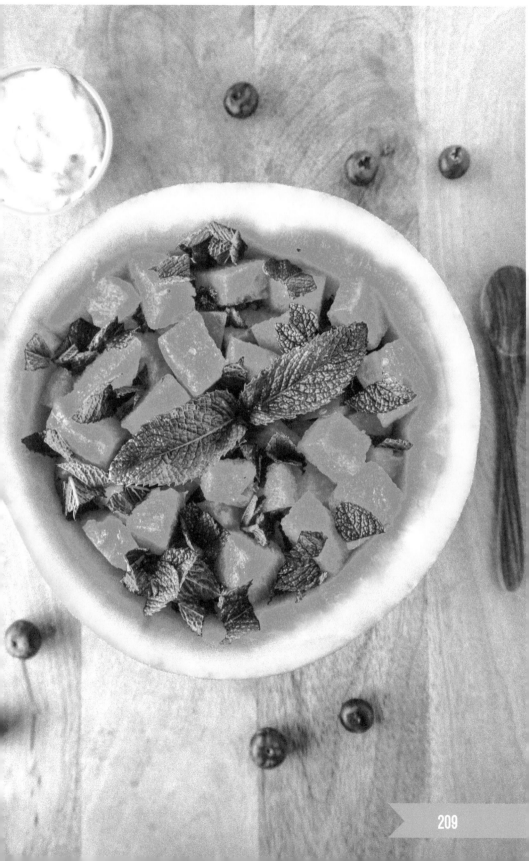

Papaya Boats

Papaya is one of my favourite foods to help heal the gut, as well as to help remove parasites from the digestive system. Whenever you visit tropical climates, make sure to eat papaya every day!

INGREDIENTS (SERVES 2)

1 small papaya
1/2 orange
1 mango (sliced)
A few blueberries
A few strawberries (sliced)
2 ripe passionfruit
Coconut yogurt to serve
Fresh mint to serve

METHOD

Slice papaya in half, lengthways and scoop out the seeds. Squeeze juice from the orange over the papaya. Fill the middle of the papaya with mango and blueberries. Top with strawberries and passionfruit, finishing with coconut yogurt and mint on top.

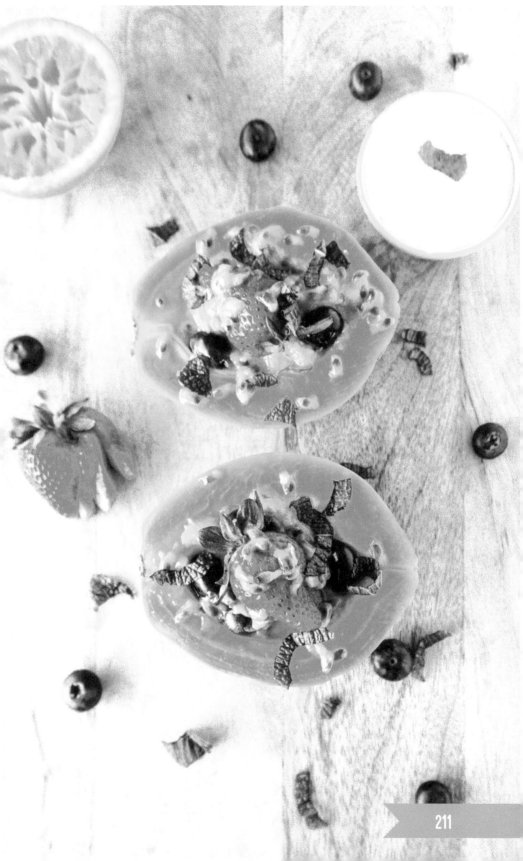

CHAPTER 27

Plant-milks + Creams

Cashew Milk

I don't use a nut bag for cashew milk because I prefer to keep all of the nutrients in it. There may be a tiny bit of sediment but just shake well before use. For the smoothest results, I use a stick blender for nut creams and milks. Although I love my blender, it can't get liquids as smooth as a stick blender. Also, the longer the nuts are soaked, the smoother the milk will be.

INGREDIENTS (MAKES 750MLS - 1 LITRE)

2 cups cashews (soaked for at least 4 hours in filtered water)
3 - 4 cups filtered water (the less water, the creamier)
1 - 2 Medjool dates or dash of pure maple syrup (optional)

METHOD

Rinse cashews thoroughly. Add to a blender, add water and dates, and blitz until smooth and creamy. Store in a sealed glass bottle for up to a week.

VARIATION

Add 1 tbsp cacao and an extra date for chocolate cashew milk.

Hemp Milk

I don't use a nut bag for hemp milk because I prefer to keep all of the nutrients in it. There may be a tiny bit of sediment but just shake well before use.

INGREDIENTS (MAKES 750ML - 1 LITRE)

3/4 cup hemp seeds (soaked in filtered water for at least 4 hours)
3 - 4 cups filtered water (the less water, the creamier)
2 Medjool dates or a dash pure maple syrup (optional)

1/2 tsp vanilla extract or powder
Small pinch pink Himalayan salt
(Optional: add 1/2 - 1 tsp of powdered purple sea moss for a super nutritious children's milk)

METHOD

Add all ingredients to a blender and blitz until smooth and creamy. Store in a sealed glass bottle for up to a week.

VARIATION

Add 1 tbsp cacao and an extra date for chocolate hemp milk.

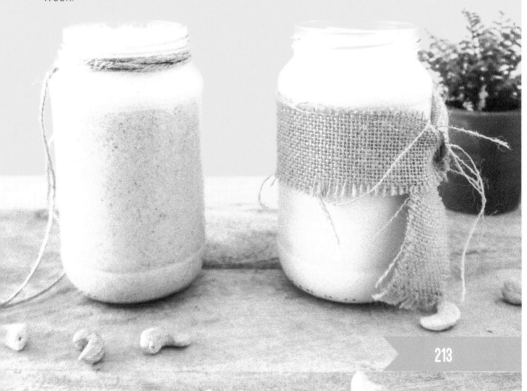

Cashew Cream

As with the plant-milks, I don't use a nut bag for cashew cream because I prefer to keep all of the nutrients in the cream. There may be a tiny bit of sediment but just shake well before use.

INGREDIENTS (MAKES APPROXIMATELY 1/2 LITRE)

2 cups cashews (soaked for at least 4 hours in filtered water)
1 cup filtered water (the less water, the creamier)

Dash of pure maple syrup
1/2 tsp vanilla extract

METHOD

Add all ingredients to a blender, gradually adding the water and checking the thickness and consistency. Blitz until smooth and creamy. Store in a sealed glass bottle for up to a week.

NOTE

When using this cream for savoury recipes, like Pumpkin Soup, omit the sweetener and vanilla, and increase water to 2 cups.

Coconut Milk

Just like coconut water, coconut milk tastes a lot better made fresh! If you can source fresh coconut, you won't regret making your own milk!

INGREDIENTS (MAKES APPROXIMATELY 1 LITRE)

3 young/green fresh coconuts
2 - 3 pitted Medjool dates (optional)

Small pinch pink Himalayan salt
1 tsp vanilla extract (optional)

METHOD

Open coconuts and pour water into a blender, using a strainer to stop any husk pieces from getting in. Scoop out the coconut jelly meat and add to the blender. Blitz until smooth and creamy. Add filtered water if needed. Store in a sealed glass bottle for up to a week.

TIP

If the coconut is young enough, you won't need to filter out any of the coconut meat. If the coconut is older or brown, then the meat will be tough. In this case, you will have to strain the fibrous chunks out with a cheesecloth or nut milk bag.

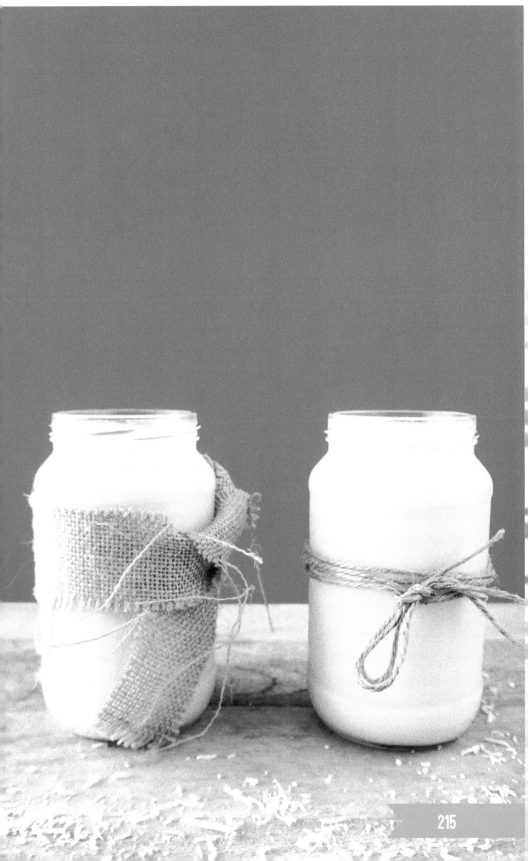

Cashew Sour Cream

Just like the plant-milks, I don't use a nut bag for this sour cream because I prefer to keep all of the nutrients in the cream. There may be a tiny bit of sediment but just shake well before use. The garlic gives this cream an Alfredo taste, which is perfect to top pizza with, instead of cheese!

INGREDIENTS (MAKES APPROXIMATELY 1/2 LITRE)

2 cups cashews (soaked for at least 4 hours in filtered water)
3/4 - 1 cup filtered water
Pinch of pink Himalayan salt
Dash apple cider vinegar
Juice of half of a lemon
1 garlic clove (optional - can use garlic powder)

METHOD

Rinse cashews thoroughly. Add all ingredients to a blender, adding water gradually. Blitz until smooth and creamy. Adjust sourness and seasoning if need. Store in a sealed glass bottle for up to a week.

(Image of recipe on page 184).

Whipped Coconut Cream

Most cans of coconut cream are different, so you may achieve a different result with each batch. The best method I have found is using a purer form of coconut cream that includes guar gum in the ingredients. Guar gum binds the fat with the rest of the cream, so the fat doesn't separate and solidify. I have tried using guar gum-free creams, but the fat separates and it becomes too solid to use, especially if put in the fridge first like most recipes suggest. Guar gum-free coconut cream works for some people, but it has never worked for me.

INGREDIENTS

1 x 15oz/400g BPA-free can coconut cream
1/2 tsp vanilla extract
Dash of pure maple syrup

METHOD

Be careful not to shake the can. Open it carefully and spoon the thick cream into a large metal bowl. Try not to scoop the coconut water out; save it for a smoothie later. Whip with a hand mixer until the cream starts to thicken, then add vanilla and maple syrup, and whip until fluffy. Whipping the cream may take about 5 minutes or so. If it doesn't form stiff peaks, put it in the fridge for about 10 - 20 minutes and then try again. Chilling the cream will help. You can also chill the metal bowl first.

Serve with Mango Buckwheat Crepes (see page 162) or Strawberry Chia Jam (see page 195).

(Image of recipe on page 163).

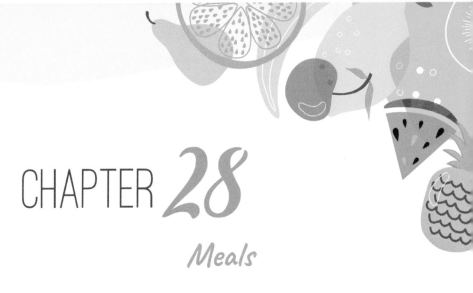

CHAPTER *28*

Meals

Sun Bowls

Sun Bowls are my go-to. Not only are they full of nutrients and lifeforce, but they're also super quick, easy, and cheap! There are so many variations that you can make so you will never get sick of them. Simply add your preferred wholegrain or cauliflower rice, your preferred legumes, and top with raw and/or steamed or roasted veggies. While these bowls don't always need a sauce, it's super easy to change it up and use Almond Satay Sauce one night, Guacamole another night, Dijon Maple another night, and Cashew Sour Cream another night. My three favourite combos are tofu or tempeh and Almond Satay Sauce, chickpeas and Dijon Maple, and black beans with Guacamole and Cashew Sour Cream for a Mexi-Sun Bowl. And if you're extra hungry, throw in some potato wedges, roast pumpkin or a Hasselback potato. Yum!

INGREDIENTS (SERVES 3)

1/2 cauliflower head (or use soaked and cooked teff or brown rice)
Salad greens
2 grated carrots
1/4 shredded red cabbage
1/2 red capsicum (chopped)
1 - 2 cucumbers (sliced)
2 cups chickpeas or black beans (soaked and cooked, or 1 x 15oz/400g BPA-free can)
Few splashes of tamari (optional)

Few dashes of cumin (optional)
Pink Himalayan salt
Black Cracked Pepper
Preferred oil to cook with

TO SERVE

Almond Satay Sauce (see page 193)
Cashew Sour Cream (see page 216)
Dijon Maple Dressing (see page 194)
Guacamole (see page 185)

METHOD

To make the cauliflower rice, wash the cauliflower, chop into several pieces, and place into a food processor. If using a blender, chop the cauliflower into smaller pieces and use the chop function. Process cauliflower until it resembles rice.

Add cauliflower to a hot pan and sauté. Season and add a touch of cumin, if preferred. Sauté until cauliflower is cooked.

At the same time, sauté the legumes and season. Add tamari to the legumes, if desired.

Add cauliflower rice to a bowl and build the Sun Bowl. Add salad greens, cabbage, legumes, cucumber, capsicum and then top with your preferred sauce. Easy!

VARIATIONS

Swap cauliflower rice for brown rice, teff, buckwheat spaghetti, or lentil pasta.

TIP

If using teff it is best soaked for 8 - 24 hours before being cooked. Use a cheesecloth to strain once ready.

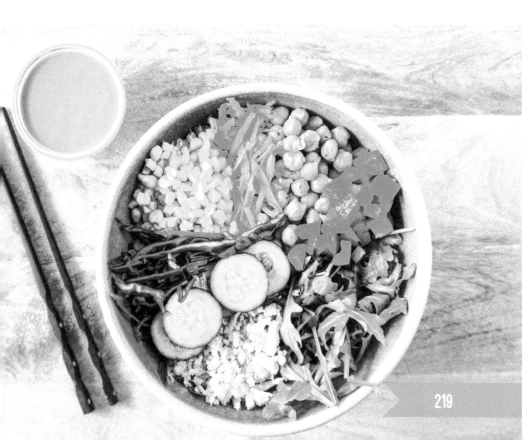

Raw Pad Thai

This is our favourite way to eat sea vegetables. You can have fun with this recipe and add so many different ingredients, like cucumber and cherry tomatoes as well. You can also switch up the nuts and use cashews, peanuts or almonds, and use almond butter, tahini, or peanut butter for the sauce. And you can change up the noodles with zucchini or carrot noodles. Enjoy!

INGREDIENTS (SERVES 3 - 4)

For the noodles

1 packet of kelp noodles
2 cups red cabbage (shredded)
1 red capsicum (thinly sliced)
1 large carrot (grated)
2 - 3 large handfuls of salad greens
1/2 cup cashews or peanuts
(roasted or activated)
Handful chopped shallots
(scallions/green onions)
1/2 cup fresh mint
(ripped, not chopped)

For the sauce

1/2 cup almond butter (can
use tahini or peanut butter)
2 to 3 tbsp tamari
1 tbsp pure maple syrup
(or 2 - 3 Medjool dates)
1/4 cup apple cider vinegar
2 - 3 tsp fresh lemon or lime juice
1 tbsp ginger
1 garlic clove
1/8 cup olive oil (can replace
with water if preferred)
Approximately 1/8 - 1/4 cup filtered
water (to reach desired consistency)
Dash of olive oil for the noodles

METHOD

Soak kelp noodles in filtered water for about 15 minutes.

Add salad ingredients to a large bowl. Add all sauce ingredients to a blender (or stick blender beaker) and blend until smooth and creamy. Adjust to suit tastes. Drain the noodles and toss with oil and add to salad. Pour sauce over the noodles and combine well, making sure all of the noodles are covered. Top with chopped nuts, shallots, and mint, then serve.

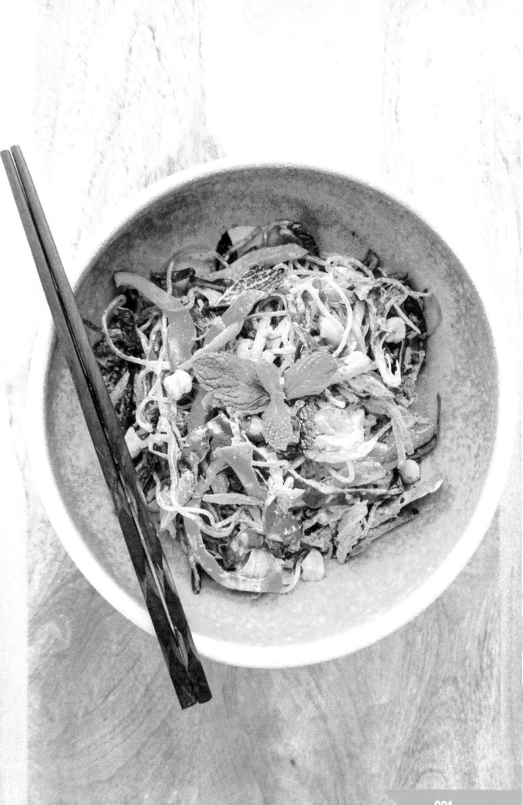

Potato and Chickpea Curry

This is the perfect mild curry for pregnancy. I absolutely love Indian food, but it doesn't contain enough vegetables for my liking. As you will see, when I make curries or dahl, I always add extra veggies to these dishes. Leafy green veggies, beans, and cauliflower are my usual go-tos.

INGREDIENTS (SERVES 4)

4 - 6 Desiree potatoes
1 Spanish onion (peeled and sliced)
3 cloves garlic (diced)
2 tsp garam masala
3 tsp ground turmeric
3 tsp ground cumin
2 - 3 tbsp grated ginger
Pinch pink Himalayan salt
4 tomatoes (diced)
1 cup filtered water

3 - 4 cups chickpeas (soaked and cooked) or 2 x 15 oz/400g BPA-free cans
1 cup cashews (optional)
2 cups green beans (sliced into quarters)
2 cups cauliflower
3 cups chopped kale (stalks removed)
1 x 15 oz/400g can coconut milk
Additional 2 cups filtered water
Preferred oil to cook with

METHOD

Peel, chop, and steam or boil potatoes in salted water for about 15 minutes, or until cooked. Drain and allow potatoes to steam in the pot for a few minutes.

To a large pot, add onion and sauté until it becomes clear. Add spices, garlic, ginger, and seasoning, and sauté for a few minutes to activate the spices.

Add diced tomatoes and simmer for 5 minutes. Add 1 cup of filtered water, cauliflower, green beans, chickpeas and cashews and simmer for another 5 - 10 minutes. Add potatoes, then add kale and stir. Add coconut milk and 1 cup of additional water, if needed, and simmer for 10 minutes. Add another cup of water if needed. Stir before serving.

Serve with brown rice and Besan Flatbread (see pages 182) or Besan Wraps (see page 180), and sprinkle hemp seeds, chopped cashews or slivered almonds over the top to add good fats.

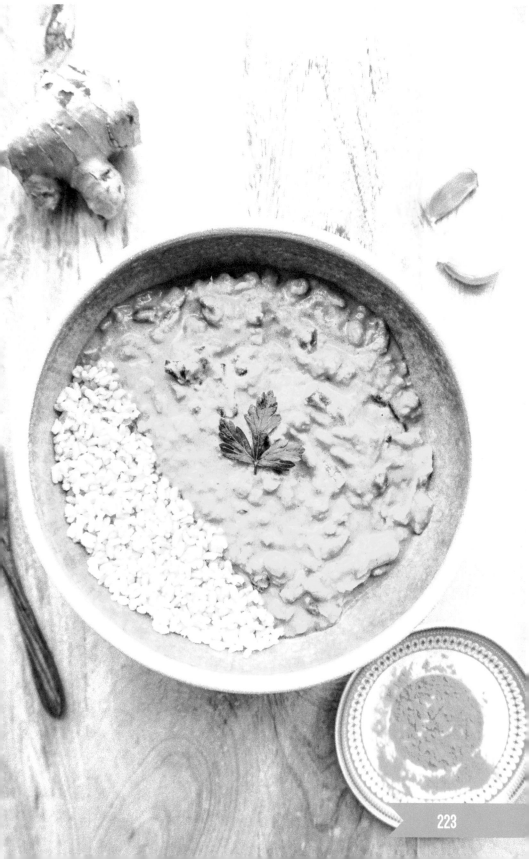

Green Bean and Kale Dahl

This dahl is mild and perfect for pregnancy. Because the lentils have been soaked overnight, they won't take too long to cook.

INGREDIENTS (SERVES 4)

3 cups red lentils (soaked overnight)
Approximately 6 cups filtered water
4 Desiree potatoes
(chopped and cooked)
1 Spanish onion (peeled and sliced)
2 tsp garam masala
3 tsp ground turmeric
3 tsp ground cumin
3 tbsp grated ginger
3 garlic cloves (diced)
Pinch pink Himalayan salt

4 tomatoes (diced)
2 - 3 cups green beans
(sliced into quarters)
3 cups chopped kale
(stalks removed)
1/2 15oz/400g BPA-free
can coconut milk
2 cups filtered water (if needed)
Preferred oil to cook with

METHOD

To a large pot, add lentils and a pinch of salt and cover with water and cook. If foam appears along the top of the water, scoop it out and empty into the sink.

To a large hot fry pan, add onion and sauté until it becomes translucent. Add spices, garlic, ginger, and seasoning, and sauté for a few minutes to activate the spices. Add diced tomatoes and simmer for 5 minutes.

When the lentils are cooked, empty some of the water out, and add the tomato and spice mix to the large pot. Then add the potatoes. Stir and simmer. Add green beans and simmer for another 5 minutes. Add kale and stir. Lastly, add coconut milk and stir. Simmer for another 10 minutes.

Serve with brown rice, and/or Besan Flatbread (see pages 182) or Besan Wraps (see page 180), and sprinkle hemp seeds, chopped cashews or slivered almonds over the top to add good fats.

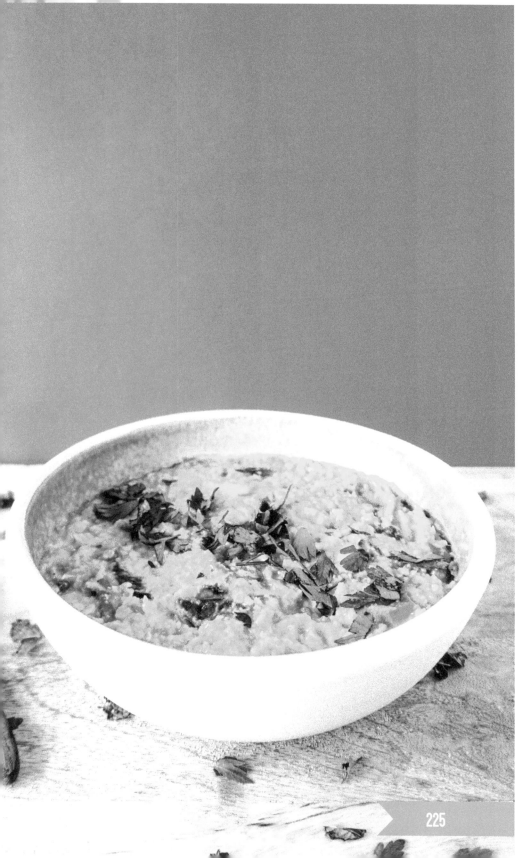

Mango, Roasted Macadamia and Nut Feta Salad

This salad is my absolute favourite, and it's so basic and super easy to make. I eat a huge bowl by itself or served as a side salad. The trick to this salad is to use the mango juice as a dressing!

INGREDIENTS (SERVE 4)

Bowl of salad greens
Punnet of grape or cherry tomatoes (halved)
2 avocados
1 mango
1/2 - 1 Spanish onion (thinly sliced)
1 cup halved macadamias (or cashews)
1/2 cup feta (I use macadamia nut feta)

METHOD

Preheat oven to 160C/320F. Spread nuts on a baking tray lined with parchment paper and bake for 5 minutes, or until golden.

Add washed salad greens to a large bowl. Add onion, tomatoes, avocado and mango cheeks and squeeze the juice and pulp from the seed over the salad greens. Add cooled nuts and top with feta.

This salad is perfect for a Vegan BBQ, to eat on its own, or to serve with Veggie Pizza Skewers (see page 240), grilled corn, and/or potato wedges.

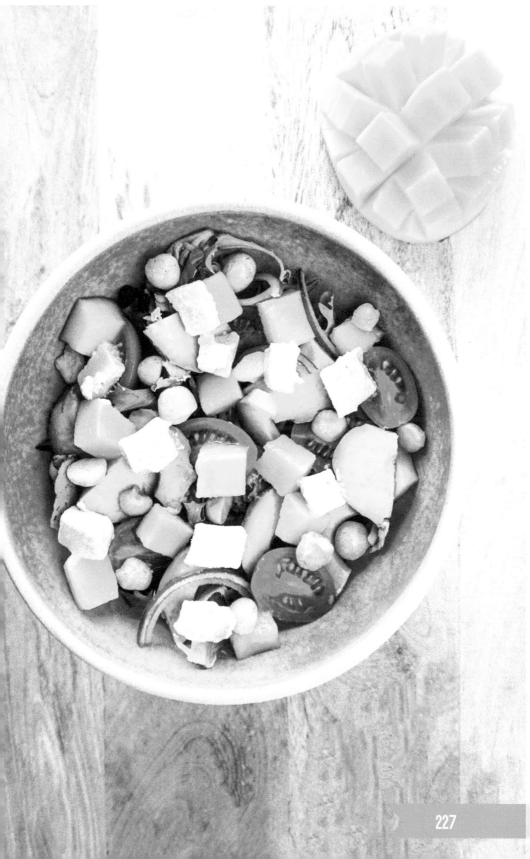

Pulled Oyster Mushroom Baguettes

I absolutely love this dish! Oyster mushrooms are a wholefood that are high in protein, fiber, iron, zinc, potassium, phosphorus, selenium, calcium, folate (B9), vitamins B1, B3, B5 and B12, and vitamin C and vitamin D. You can use regular Pearl Oyster mushrooms or King Oyster mushrooms, or you can use jackfruit. The marinade should be enough for about 800g of jackfruit. Coconut oil solidifies so if you opt for coconut oil, don't put the marinade in the fridge, and let the mushrooms return to room temperature before adding them to the marinade. Also, be mindful if the weather is cold. The mushrooms don't need to marinate for too long as they're super spongy and soak up the marinade easily. If using jackfruit, marinate for at least 2 hours. I find it easiest to marinate in an airtight container as it's easy to shake and turn upside down. Paprika has a spicy kick to it so try 1 teaspoon at first. I use sourdough baguettes but use whichever rolls you prefer.

INGREDIENTS (SERVES 2)

2 tbsp tamari sauce (salt-reduced)
2 tbsp coconut sugar
2 tbsp olive oil or melted coconut oil
1 - 2 tsp paprika
300g oyster mushrooms
1 sourdough baguette
Avocado
Shredded romaine (cos) lettuce

METHOD

Add tamari, coconut sugar, oil and paprika to an airtight container with a lid. Mix well. Wash, dry and slice mushrooms lengthways. Add mushrooms to the container, put the lid on, and shake well until mushrooms are completely covered.

To a hot pan, add mushrooms and the marinade and sauté until the marinade reduces. Should take about 5 - 10 minutes. While the mushrooms are cooking, slice the baguette in half, lengthways, and grill in the oven for about 5 minutes or until golden brown. Once the mushrooms are cooked, place them on a wooden chopping board and use 2 forks to 'pull' the mushrooms.

Spread avocado on the toasted baguette, add romaine, then top with mushrooms. Serve with a side salad.

VARIATION

Use the marinade to marinate chickpeas and toss in a roasted pumpkin and rocket salad.

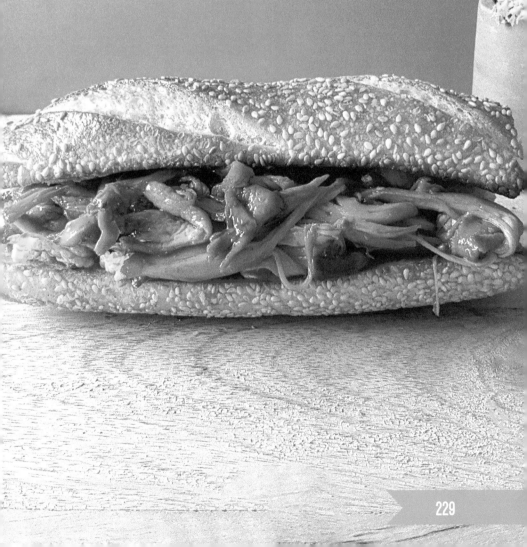

Sprouted Lentil Burgers

These lentil patties are another one of our favourites. The lentils and garlic are the heroes of this dish, and they even keep meat-eaters happy too! For a treat, melt (clean) vegan cheese on top and make a cheeseburger.

INGREDIENTS (MAKES 5 LARGE PATTIES)

4 cups sprouted beluga lentils (can use overnight soaked lentils)
Large pinch pink Himalayan salt
3 garlic cloves
Large handful of fresh oregano (optional)
Approximately 1/4 to 1/2 cup buckwheat flour.
2 tbsp tamari
Preferred oil to cook with
Sweet Potato Wraps (see page 186), or preferred sourdough/rolls to serve

METHOD

Throw all ingredients into a food processor or into a powerful blender. If using a blender, you will need to stop and scrape down the sides every few seconds. Don't blend too much and leave some texture. The mixture should stick together but should not be dry or crumbly. Taste the mixture and see if it needs any more pink salt or herbs.

Roll into balls for patties or roll into small balls for lentil falafel.

To a hot pan, add patties and cook for 5 minutes on each side, or until golden brown.

Serve with an array of fresh salad vegetables in a Sweet Potato Wrap (see page 186) or preferred bread. Top with Avocado Mayo (see page 192) and/or Tomato Relish (see page 190).

TIP

If you want to, only add 3 cups of the lentils to the processor and add the other cup of lentils to the mixing bowl, so you have a mixture of blended and whole lentils.

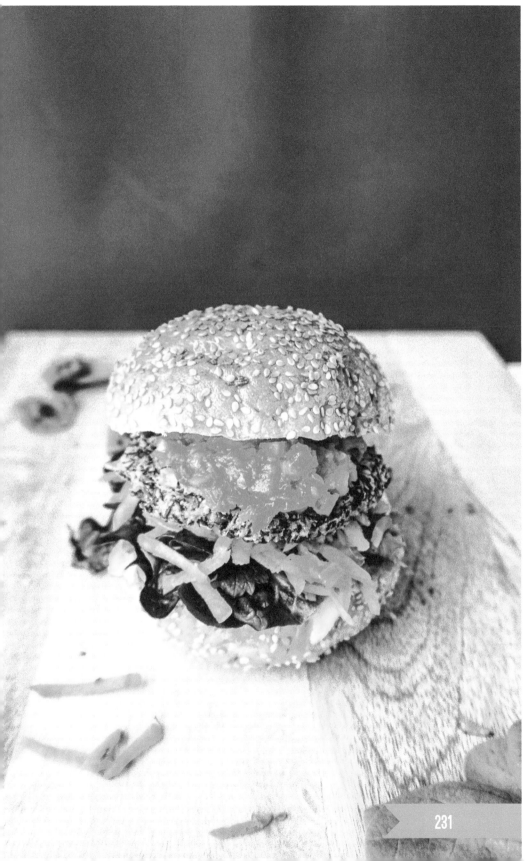

Chickpea and Sweet Potato Burger Patties

These patties can be made with or without the sweet potato. The sweet potato gives these patties a softer texture with a hint of sweetness. Without the sweet potato, the chickpeas are the hero giving it a more savoury flavour.

INGREDIENTS (MAKES 8)

1/2 large sweet potato
2 cups chickpeas (soaked and cooked) or 1 x 15 oz/400g BPA-free can
Handful chopped shallots (scallions/green onions) or fresh parsley
1/2 - 1 cup buckwheat flour

1/2 - 1 tsp ground cumin
1/2 tsp paprika
1/2 tsp turmeric
1 tbsp flaxmeal
Pinch pink Himalayan salt
Pinch black cracked pepper

METHOD

Peel and chop sweet potato and steam/boil in salted water. When cooked, drain and steam dry in the pot. Allow to cool.

In a food processor or in a large bowl with a stick blender, process chickpeas and pulse to break them down. Don't over-process them in order to leave some texture. Add potato, flour, flaxmeal, seasoning and spices and hand mix with a fork. Fold in shallots or parsley. The mixture should form a sticky dough. It should have some stickiness otherwise the patties will dry out. Roll into large balls and add to a hot pan. Flatten and cook for 3 - 5 minutes on each side, or until golden brown.

Serve as a burger with Tomato Relish (see page 190), or with a huge side salad and grilled corn.

VARIATION

Change it up and replace the chickpeas with black beans or roll the mixture up into small balls to make veggie balls.

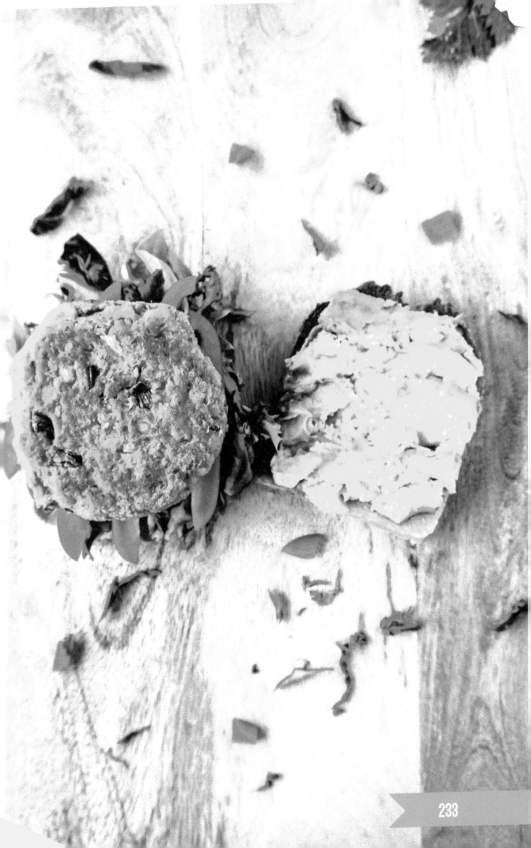

Raw Alfredo

I love how light and easy zucchini noodles, zoodles, are. If you don't have a spiralizer, you can use a standard potato peeler to create pappardelle-type zoodles. You can also add half zoodles and half seaweed noodles instead.

INGREDIENTS (SERVES 3 - 4)

4 - 6 zucchini (peeled and spiralized)
2 cups cashews (soaked overnight in filtered water)
3/4 - 1 cup filtered water
Pinch of pink Himalayan salt
Pinch black pepper
Dash apple cider vinegar
Juice of half of a lemon
1 garlic clove

METHOD

Blend cashews, garlic, seasoning, apple cider vinegar, and lemon juice until thick, smooth and creamy, adding water gradually. Add more water if needed. You may need to scrape down the sides a few times, but don't add too much water, as the sauce will thin out once it's added to the zucchini noodles.

Pour sauce over zoodles. Mix in freshly chopped shallots and serve immediately.

Serve with a green side salad, freshly sautéed chickpeas and/or potato wedges.

TIP

When working with zucchini noodles, the water content can make the sauce runny. If this is an issue, drain the zoodles in a strainer before adding the sauce. I usually place a cup under the strainer and push the noodles down, catching the water in the cup. Drink the nutrient-dense water instead of tipping it down the sink.

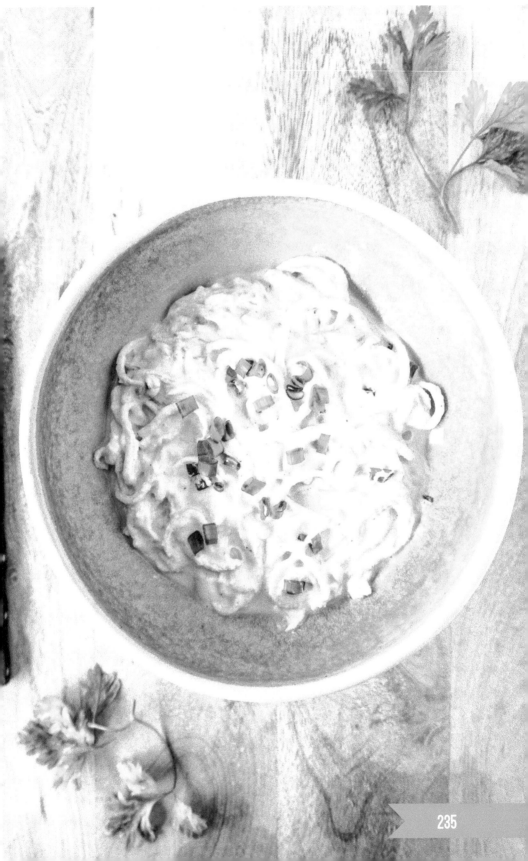

Lentil Bolognese

A hearty yet light and nutritious meal that also uses zoodles. You can swap out the zoodles for legume or wholegrain pasta as well. If you find lentils tough to digest, pre-cook them in salted water first, making sure not to overcook them.

INGREDIENTS (SERVES 3 - 4)

6 large zucchinis (peeled and spiralized)
2 cups green or brown lentils (soaked overnight)
2 garlic cloves (crushed)
1 tbsp tomato paste
1 Spanish onion (diced)
1 carrot (grated)
6 tomatoes (finely diced) or use passata instead (glass bottle, not from a can)

1 - 2 tbsp tamari
1 - 2 cups filtered water
2 cups mushrooms (sliced)
2 tbsp dried oregano or thyme
1 tsp onion powder (optional)
1 tsp garlic powder (optional)
Handful fresh oregano or basil
Pinch pink Himalayan salt
Preferred oil to cook with

METHOD

Drain and rinse the lentils. Set aside.

Add oil to a hot pan and sauté onion until it becomes translucent. Add the garlic and stir. Mix in the tomato paste, tomatoes, lentils, tamari, dried herbs, and water. Season, stir well, and simmer.

When the lentils are nearly cooked, add the carrot and sauté. In a separate pan, sauté mushrooms with garlic and a dash of tamari, and season. To the lentil mixture, add fresh herbs, garlic powder and onion powder and mix through. Simmer and adjust to suit tastes. Fold in sautéed mushrooms. I prefer to add the mushrooms at the end to keep them flavoursome. You can skip this step and add the mushrooms when you add the carrots.

Add zucchini noodles to bowls and top with Bolognese sauce. Sprinkle with extra herbs to serve. If you have a clean vegan cheese, sprinkle some on top!

TIP

You can make this sauce ahead of time and keep it in the freezer until ready to use.

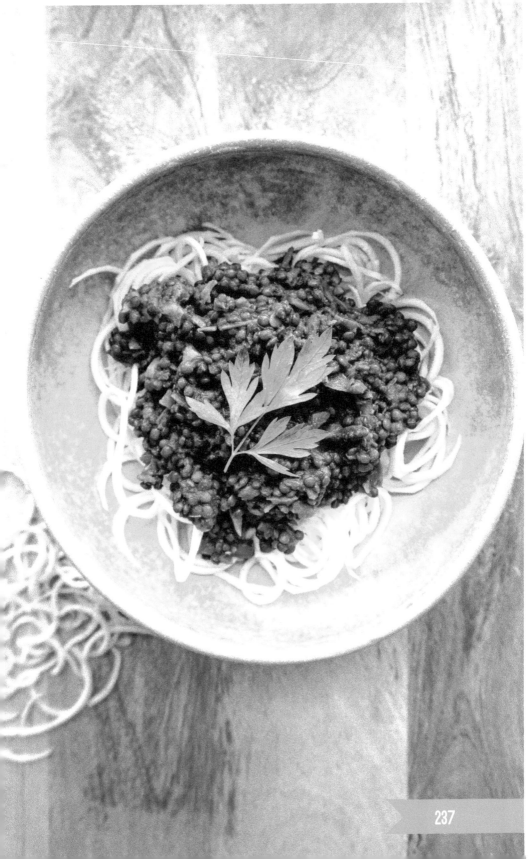

Tijuana Sweet Potato Boats
+ 3 Alternative Recipes

Mexi-anything keeps most people happy, and it's super versatile. Using the same ingredients, you can make Sweet Potato Boats, Nachos, Tortillas, and Mexi-Sun Bowls.

INGREDIENTS

2 large sweet potatoes
4 - 5 cups black beans
(soaked and cooked) or 2 x 15
oz/400g BPA-free cans
Pinch pink Himalayan salt
Black cracked pepper
Dash tamari sauce
Large pinch cumin and/
or smoked paprika
Preferred oil to cook with

1 cup red cabbage (shredded)
2 tomatoes (diced)
1 fresh corn cob (kernels cut off)
1 cup red capsicum/
bell pepper (diced)
Handful of chopped shallots
(scallions/green onions)
or fresh parsley
Guacamole (see page 185)
Cashew sour cream (see page 216)

METHOD

Preheat oven to 200C/392F. Scrub sweet potato, leaving the skin on. If you're using large potatoes, slice sweet potato lengthways in half. Otherwise, you can keep them whole and pierce a few holes in each potato. Season and drizzle with oil and bake for about 45 minutes or until tender and cooked through. Sweet potato will roast perfectly without oil, so you can omit the oil if preferred.

While the potatoes are baking, prepare the beans, guacamole, and sour cream.

To a hot pan add garlic and sauté, then add black beans. Stir and add tamari, seasoning, cumin, and paprika. If mixture begins to dry out, add a dash of water and stir.

In a separate pan, stir-fry corn and season.

When the sweet potato is cooked, remove from the oven and allow to cool. If using halved potatoes, season and use the back of a fork to push the sweet potato down. If using whole potatoes, slice lengthways straight down the middle and fold open.

Stuff with beans, red cabbage, capsicum, tomato, corn, guacamole, and sour cream. Sprinkle with fresh herbs.

ALTERNATIVE RECIPES

Replace the black beans with pan-seared mushrooms and use in this recipe or in Home-Made Tortillas (see page 184).

Replace the sweet potato with corn chips or home-made baked sweet potato chips and make epic nachos!

Replace the sweet potato with salad greens and brown rice or cauli-rice to make a Tijuana Sun Bowl. Yum!

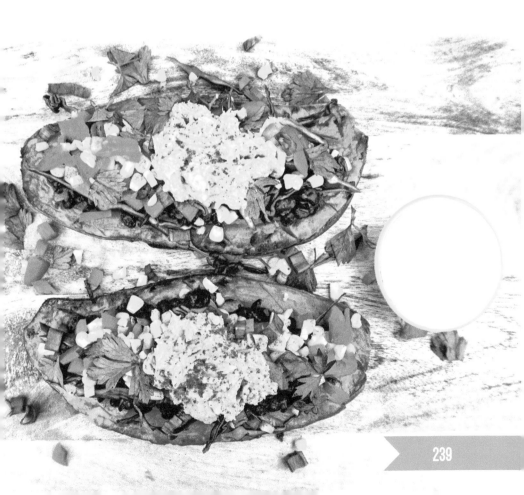

Veggie Pizza Skewers

Perfect for the Vegan BBQ, these pizza skewers are simple to make and taste amazing!

INGREDIENTS (MAKES 15)

15 cherry or grape tomatoes
1/2 pineapple
2 zucchinis
15 whole button mushrooms
2 red capsicum

FOR THE MARINADE

1 tbsp pure maple syrup
or date syrup
1 tbsp dried oregano
or Italian herbs
2 tbsp tamari
Wooden or steel skewers

METHOD

Chop pineapple and capsicum into medium-sized pieces, and slice zucchini into circles, about 1.5cm thick. Add to a large bowl with whole button mushrooms and tomatoes.

In a small separate bowl, add maple syrup, herbs, and tamari and mix. Adjust to suit tastes and add to veggies. Using your hands, mix and coat thoroughly. Leave to marinate for at least one hour.

Thread veggies and fruit onto skewers, making sure to thread the zucchini through the skin so it doesn't break and fall off. If there is any leftover marinade, pour it over the skewers, and BBQ or bake until veggies are tender.

Serve on a bed of rocket greens with marinated and grilled tempeh or tofu, grilled corn, smashed avocado and brown rice. Or add the tempeh to the skewers.

TIP

If baking and using wooden skewers, soak the skewers in water for a few hours beforehand so they do not burn.

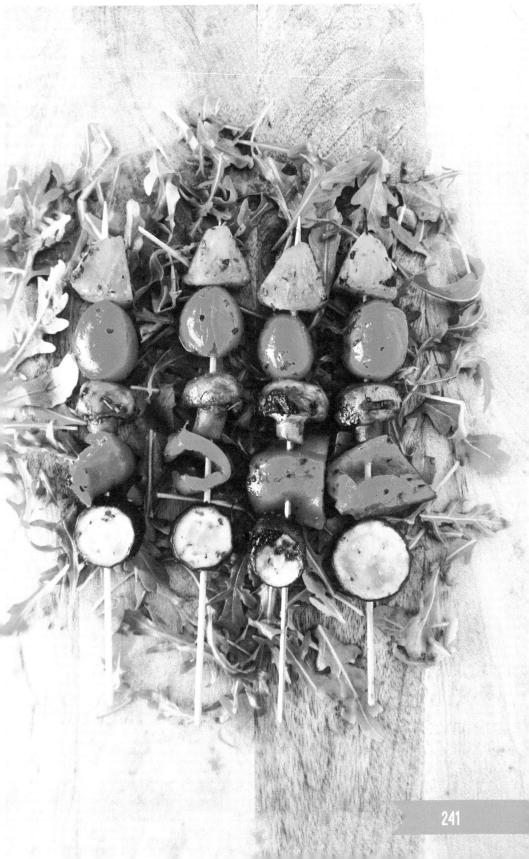

Lentil Ramen

This ramen is a Winter favourite! It's warming, soothing and doesn't take long to make. The lentils shouldn't take long to cook because they have been soaked overnight.

INGREDIENTS (SERVES 3 - 4)

3 large zucchinis for zoodles (can substitute with buckwheat ramen noodles)
3 cups green lentils (soaked overnight)
8 - 10 cups filtered water
2 organic carrots (thinly sliced)
1/2 broccoli

1 baby bok choy
4 tbsp tamari
2 cloves garlic
1 - 2 tbsp grated ginger
Handful of chopped shallots (scallions/green onions)
Pinch pink Himalayan salt
Preferred oil to cook with

METHOD

Rinse lentils thoroughly. In a large pot, cook the lentils in about 4 cups of water and lightly salt. Keep an eye on the water level, the lentils should always be covered in water. Add more water if you need to and be sure not to overcook them.

While the lentils are cooking, spiralize the zucchinis. If you don't like the raw skin taste, peel the zucchinis and keep the peels for later. You will have some leftovers from making zoodles, so chop these up and save these as well.

In a hot pan, stir-fry the vegetables adding zucchini skins last, being sure not to overcook the vegetables.

The lentils should be ready now. You will be making the broth in the lentil pot with the lentils, so keep the water and lentils in there. Add 2 cups of water to the lentils and allow to heat. Add tamari, garlic, ginger, and pink Himayalan salt. Add as much water as you need to and keep taste testing as you do this. Once you are happy with the broth, you are ready to plate.

In a deep bowl, add some of the zoodles, then top with stir-fried vegetables. Top with lentils and broth. To finish, top with shallots (and chilli after pregnancy).

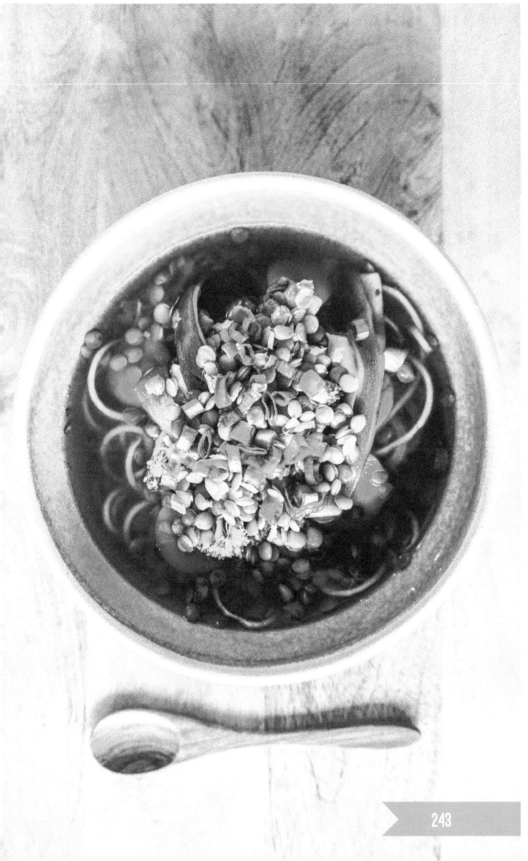

Lentil, Mushroom & Spinach Shepherds Pie

I like to keep the mushrooms and the lentils as the heroes of this dish, so I don't add too many ingredients, but you can add fresh or dried thyme or oregano once the lentil mixture is ready. I keep the lentil stock and use it to sauté the vegetables. The onion powder and garlic powder are optional, but I like to add them for extra flavour. I also sprinkle some on top of the mashed potato before baking the pie.

INGREDIENTS (SERVES 6)

2 cups green lentils (soaked overnight)
2 garlic cloves (diced)
1 large carrot (grated)
1 - 2 zucchinis (finely chopped)
3 - 4 cups mushrooms (sliced)
1 - 2 tsp onion powder (optional)
1 - 2 tsp garlic powder (optional)
2 - 3 tbsp tamari
Pink Himalayan salt, to taste
Cracked black pepper
1/2 - 1 cup filtered water (or lentil stock)
2 large handfuls of baby spinach
5 - 6 Desiree potatoes or 2 large sweet potatoes (cooked and mashed)
Sesame seeds and hemp seeds (optional)
Preferred oil to cook with
1 cup of filtered water (if needed)

METHOD

Rinse the lentils and cook in filtered water until almost soft. This shouldn't take too long because the lentils have been soaked. Try not to cook all the way through so you don't cook the lentils twice. Preheat oven to 200C/390F.

While the lentils are cooking, in a large pan sauté garlic and then add mushrooms and a dash of tamari. Remove mushrooms from pan. To the pan, add oil, carrot and zucchini. If the pan is dry, add some water/stock to sauté the vegetables and to help create a sauce. Add the onion powder and garlic powder and stir through. Heat through and add the lentils and combine. Add more water if needed, add tamari, and season. Take off the heat, add spinach and mushrooms, and stir through. Taste and adjust flavours. I prefer to add the mushrooms in at the end to keep the mushrooms flavoursome. You can skip this step if you prefer.

Add lentil mixture to a baking dish. Top with mashed potatoes and season. If you have a preferred (and clean) vegan cheese that you use, grate and add to the top of the pie. I like to sprinkle onion powder, garlic powder, Himalayan salt, hemp seeds and sesame seeds on top before baking. Bake for about 15 minutes, or until golden brown on top. When ready, remove from the oven and allow to cool.

VARIATION

Use the lentil mixture from the Lentil Bolognese (see page 236) for a tomato and herb shepherd's pie. Yum!

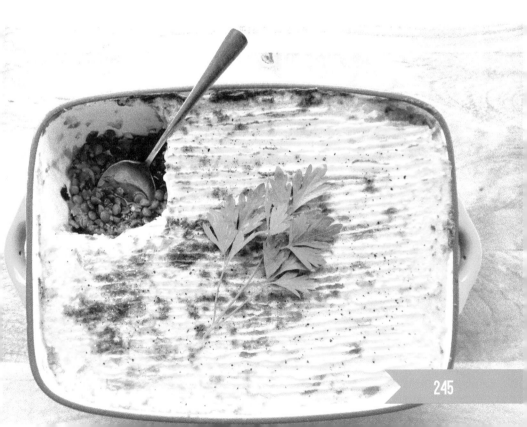

Creamy Pumpkin Soup

This soup is super simple, and it tastes better than any other pumpkin soup I've ever tried. The secret is to let the pumpkin be the hero of the dish, so don't hide its flavour behind apples and spices. Plus, the onions also act as a sweetener. You can use any plant-milk, but I prefer to use fresh cashew cream as its richness helps make the soup, and it adds good fats to the dish. If onions make you gassy, soak the peeled onions in filtered water for at least 3 hours before dicing.

INGREDIENTS (SERVES 3 - 4)

1/2 large ripe Kent pumpkin (ripe Kents have a dark orange flesh)
2 Spanish onions (diced)
Cashew cream (see page 214)
Large pinch pink Himalayan salt
Black cracked pepper
Plant-milk or filtered water if needed

METHOD

Peel pumpkin and steam or boil in salted water until cooked. If time permits, bake the pumpkin while in its skin instead. When the pumpkin is cooked, drain thoroughly. If baking, scoop the pumpkin out of the skin and put aside to cool.

In a large pot, add Spanish onion and sauté until browned and sweet. Add pumpkin to the pot, and then add the cashew cream. Purée with a stick blender, and then heat if needed. If consistency is too thick, add plant-milk or filtered water.

Serve with fresh and/or steamed greens, Besan Flatbread (see page 182) or your favourite crusty bread.

VARIATION

After you have tried this recipe, you will notice that it has a mild cheezy flavour, which is perfect for home-made mac'n'cheeze. Add less liquid so the soup becomes a thick cheezy sauce. Toss in garlic and onion powder for flavour. Yum!

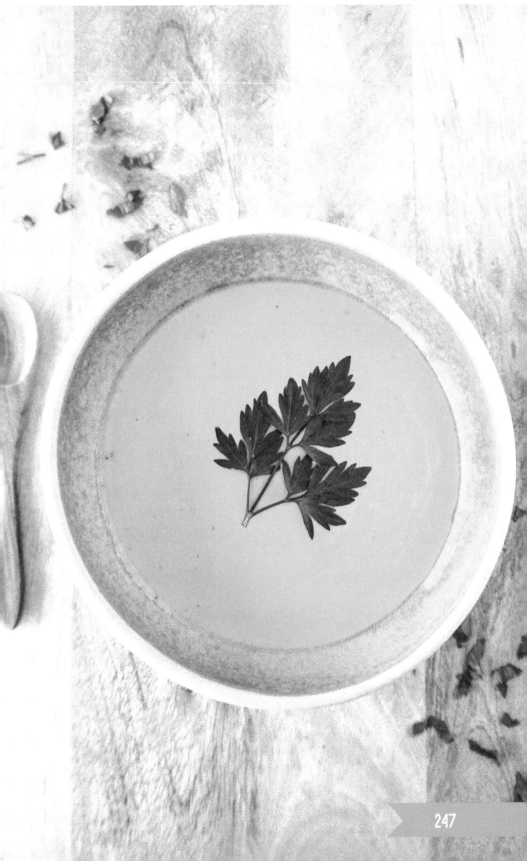

Curried Lentil Veggie Soup

A hearty and nutritious soup for those cooler months! Use chick peas if you do not have lentils.

INGREDIENTS

1 Spanish onion
2 cloves garlic
1 - 2 tbsp grated ginger
2 - 3 tsp ground turmeric (optional)
2 tbsp curry powder
3 Desiree potatoes (chopped)
1/4 Kent pumpkin (chopped)
4 cups green lentils (soaked overnight)
1/4 cauliflower (chopped)
1 carrot (chopped)
Greens, such as bok choy and broccoli (chopped)
Large pinch pink Himalayan salt
Large pink black cracked pepper
4 tbsp tamari sauce
Approximately 2 litres/8 cups filtered water or fresh veggie stock

METHOD

Drain and rinse lentils.

In a large soup pot, sauté onion until transparent, and then add garlic and stir. Add ginger, curry powder, turmeric, salt, pepper, and potato, and sauté for about 5 minutes. Add pumpkin and stir for another 5 minutes. Add water and tamari. Bring to the boil, add lentils, and simmer.

When the potato is almost cooked, add the carrot and cauliflower. Simmer for another 5 minutes, then add the rest of the veggies and simmer until vegetables are tender. Adjust seasoning and water if needed.

Serve with Besan Flatbread (see page 182) or a crusty sourdough roll. Yum!

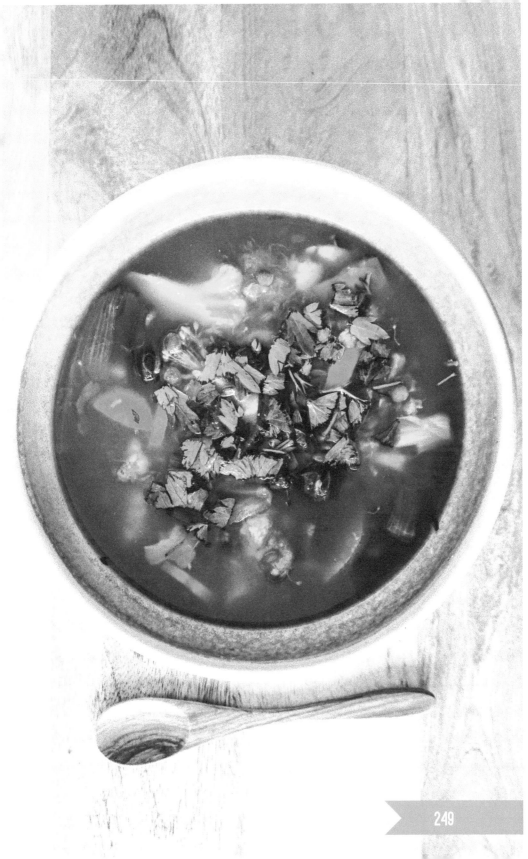

Creamy Potato & Leek Soup

This soup is super simple, and it tastes better than any other potato and leek soup I've ever tried. As with the pumpkin soup, the secret is to let the potato and leek be the heroes of the dish, so don't hide its flavour behind too many ingredients. You can use any plant-milk or fresh stock, but I prefer to use a blend of plant-milk and cashew cream as its richness helps make the soup, and the cashews add good fats.

INGREDIENTS (SERVES 4)

6 Desiree potatoes (peeled and chopped)
2 medium leeks (sliced)
3-4 cups filtered water or fresh veggie stock
Cashew cream (see page 214)
Large pinch pink Himayalan salt (to taste)
Large pinch black cracked pepper
Preferred oil to cook with

METHOD

To a large soup pot, add oil and sauté leeks until golden. Add potato and sauté until golden brown. Season with salt and pepper. Add water or stock and cook until potato is tender.

Remove half of the potato and add the cashew cream. Blend with a stick blender and add the remaining potato back to the pot. Alternatively, you can blend all of the potatoes for a completely puréed soup. Taste and adjust seasoning.

Serve with fresh and steamed greens and beans, sourdough or Sweet Potato Flatbread (see page 186).

VARIATIONS

Add chickpeas after blending the soup for some added nutrients. Or replace the potatoes with one head of cauliflower and fresh sweet corn, for a yummy sweet corn and cauliflower soup.

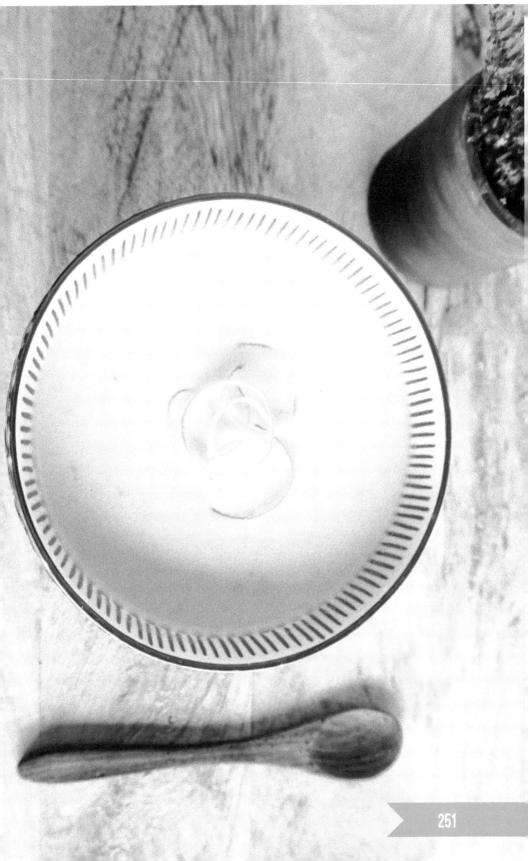

Sweet Potato, Ginger & Lemongrass Soup

I absolutely love this soup. It's thick and creamy, super easy to make, and the ginger and lemongrass are the perfect partners for sweet potato!

INGREDIENTS (SERVES 4)

4 medium sweet potatoes
2 tbsp ginger (grated)
1 stalk lemongrass (halved and bruised)
3 - 4 cups filtered water or fresh veggie stock
1 x 15 oz. can coconut milk (BPA-free can)
Preferred oil to cook with
Pink Himalayan salt
Black cracked pepper

METHOD

Preheat oven to 200C/392F. Leaving the skin on, cut sweet potato in half lengthways and place on a baking tray skin-side down. Season and drizzle with oil and bake for 40 minutes or until tender. If time doesn't permit, you can steam or boil the sweet potato, but it tastes much better baked.

While the sweet potato is baking, add coconut milk, stock/water, lemongrass, and ginger to a large soup pot and bring to the boil. When the potato is ready, remove from the oven and allow to cool. Scoop sweet potato out of the skins and add to the pot. You can remove the lemongrass, or leave it in, and blend with a stick blender until smooth and creamy. Depending on your blender, there may be fibrous chunks in the soup if you leave the lemongrass in.

Serve with hemp seeds, steamed greens and toasted sourdough.

VARIATION

For a less creamy soup, replace the coconut milk with plant-milk or fresh vegetable stock.

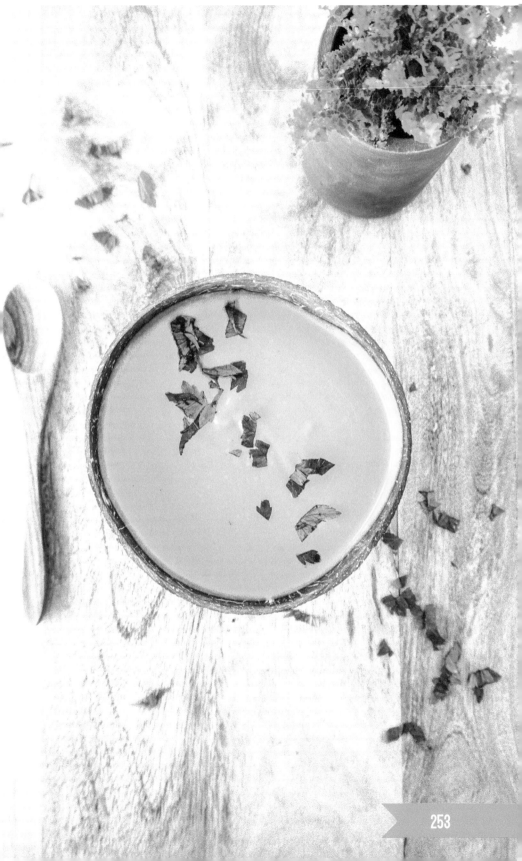

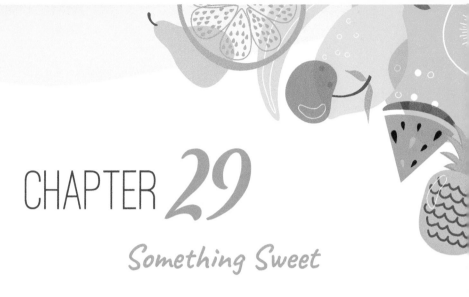

CHAPTER *29*

Something Sweet

Raw Snickerz

This snickerz is simple, tasty, and nutrient dense. It contains B-vitamins, vitamin E, magnesium, potassium, selenium, phosphorus, calcium, iron, and zinc, plus more!

FOR THE BASE

1 cup almonds or cashews
1 cup peanuts
6 - 7 Medjool dates (pitted)
Tiny pinch pink Himalayan salt
Process all ingredients until mixture sticks together and forms a dough. Add more dates if needed. Press into a lined tray as the base.

FOR THE PEANUT CARAMEL

1/2 cup pure maple syrup or date paste
1/2 cup unhulled tahini
1/4 cup coconut butter OR coconut oil (melted)
1 cup peanuts
1/2 - 1tsp vanilla extract
Tiny pinch pink Himalayan salt
Mix all ingredients together, adding butter/oil and peanuts last. Adjust sweetener/salt/vanilla if needed.
Pour on top of the peanut base and place in the fridge.

FOR THE CHOCOLATE

1 cup cacao butter
2 tbsp cacao powder
2 tbsp pure maple syrup
1/2 tsp vanilla powder or extract
1/2 tsp ground cinnamon (optional)

Peanuts to garnish

Melt cacao butter in a small saucepan or in a double boiler. Add remaining ingredients and stir until combined and velvety.

Pour chocolate on top of peanut caramel and place in the fridge to set. Add peanuts to the top before chocolate completely hardens. Leave in the fridge for a few hours before slicing. Store in an airtight container in the fridge for up to 2 weeks.

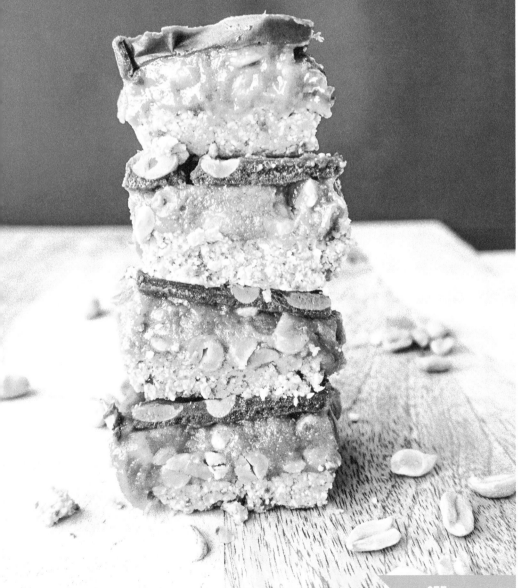

Chocnana Skewers

These are a hit at dinner parties and vegan BBQs. Served frozen, the banana coins resemble an ice cream texture, so many people don't even realize that they're eating bananas! The bananas also turn creamy if left out of the freezer for about 10 minutes before serving.

INGREDIENTS (MAKES 9 - 10)

6 bananas
1 cup cacao butter
2 tbsp cacao powder
2 tbsp pure maple syrup
1/2 tsp vanilla powder or extract
1/4 tsp ground cinnamon (optional)
Caramel from page 260 (optional)
Garnishes such as crushed freeze-dried raspberries/strawberries, shredded coconut, caramelized buckinis, or
roasted almonds or peanuts
Skewers (can use iceblock sticks)

METHOD

Peel bananas and slice into thick 3cm coins, and thread the coins on to the skewers. Thread the bananas through the sides rather than the middle. Place in the freezer.

Prepare the chocolate. Melt cacao butter in a small saucepan or in a double boiler. Add remaining ingredients. Continue stirring until mixture is smooth and creamy. Taste and adjust ingredients if needed.

When the bananas are cold or almost frozen, remove from the freezer and cover with chocolate. If the bananas are cold enough, the chocolate will begin to set instantly. Decorate with your favourite garnishes before the chocolate sets.

If the bananas aren't cold enough put them back in the freezer, otherwise you will need to double coat them. If double-coating, dip the bananas in chocolate and place the skewers back into the freezer until the chocolate is set, then cover with a second coat of chocolate. Decorate with your favourite garnishes, before the second coat sets.

My favourite combos are chocolate and crushed freeze-dried strawberries, and as pictured, chopped peanuts and shredded coconut, then drizzled with caramel sauce. If using the caramel sauce, thin out the sauce with a dash of plant-milk and gently heat in a saucepan.

Place in the freezer for about 30 minutes or until chocolate has set. Eat now or leave in the freezer and enjoy when ready!

Store in an airtight container in the freezer for 2 - 3 weeks.

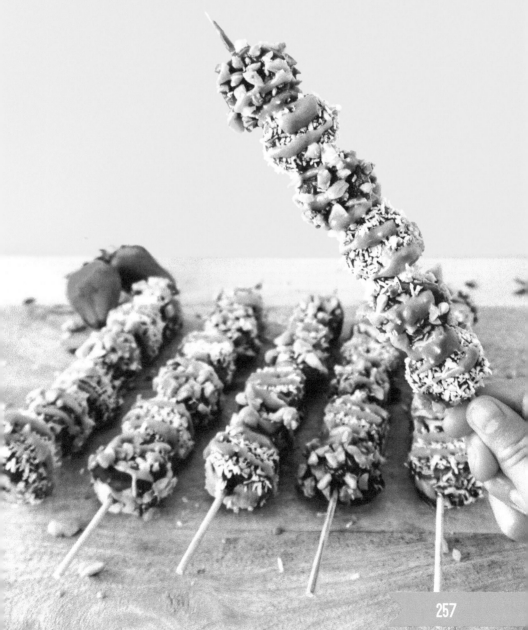

Choc-Covered Stuffed Dates

Dates are my preferred sweetener. A wholefood that's loaded with vitamins and minerals, they are perfect for those who want to watch their blood sugar levels. There are so many variations that you can do with stuffing dates, both savoury and sweet. Personally, my absolute favourite go-to dessert is dates stuffed with almond butter with a sprinkle of vanilla powder and a tiny dash of pink Himalayan salt, kept in the freezer. Yum!

INGREDIENTS

10 Medjool dates
1/4 cup almond butter or peanut butter or tahini

OPTIONAL, RAW CHOCOLATE

1/2 cup cacao butter
1 tbsp cacao powder
1 tbsp pure maple syrup
1/4 tsp vanilla powder or extract
1/4 tsp ground cinnamon (optional)

METHOD

Carefully slice the dates along the side and remove seeds. Using your fingers, carefully widen and hollow out the dates. With a teaspoon, place about 1/2 teaspoon of nut butter into the center.

If you're going to dip in chocolate, put dates in the freezer for an hour first. Line tray or a large plate with parchment paper. Prepare the chocolate. Melt cacao butter in a small saucepan or in a double boiler. Add remaining ingredients. Continue stirring until mixture is smooth and creamy.

Dip each date in the chocolate and place on a tray and put into the fridge or freezer. If the dates are cold enough, the chocolate should begin to thicken and harden immediately. If the dates aren't cold enough, you will have to do two coatings.

If not dipping in chocolate, sprinkle the tops of each date with vanilla powder and a tiny dash of pink Himalayan salt, and keep in the freezer until ready to eat. The dates and nut butter don't completely freeze, and they're super chewy.

If there is any leftover chocolate add to a bowl of nicecream.

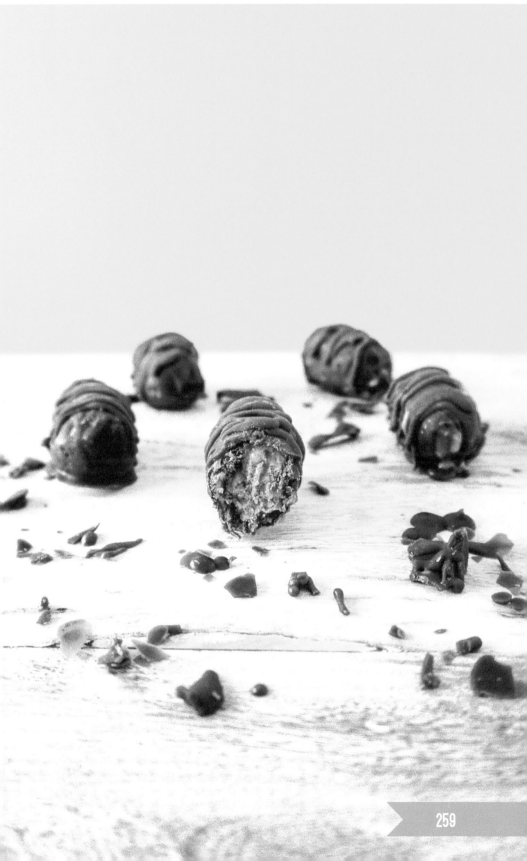

Raw Caramel Slice

A tweaked Snickerz recipe, this caramel slice is tasty and nutrient dense: including B-vitamins, vitamin E, magnesium, potassium, selenium, phosphorus, calcium, iron, and zinc, plus more!

INGREDIENTS

For the Base

1 cup almonds or cashews
1 cup shredded coconut
6 - 7 Medjool dates (pitted)
Tiny pinch pink Himalayan salt
Process all ingredients until mixture sticks together and forms a dough. Add more dates if needed. Press into a lined tray as the base.

For the Caramel

1/2 cup of pure maple syrup or date paste
1/2 cup unhulled tahini
1/4 cup coconut butter OR coconut oil (melted)
1/2 - 1 tsp vanilla extract
Tiny pinch pink Himalayan salt

Mix all ingredients together, adding butter/oil last. Adjust sweetener/salt/vanilla if needed. Pour on top of base and place in the fridge.

FOR THE CHOCOLATE

1 cup cacao butter
2 tbsp cacao powder
2 tbsp pure maple syrup
1/2 tsp vanilla powder or extract
1/2 tsp ground cinnamon (optional)

Melt cacao butter in a small saucepan or in a double boiler. Add remaining ingredients and stir until thick and creamy. Pour on top of caramel and place in the fridge to set. Leave in the fridge or freezer for a few hours before slicing. Store in an airtight container in the fridge for up to 2 weeks.

TIP

I usually put some of the caramel aside to use in Snickerz Nicecream (see page 274).

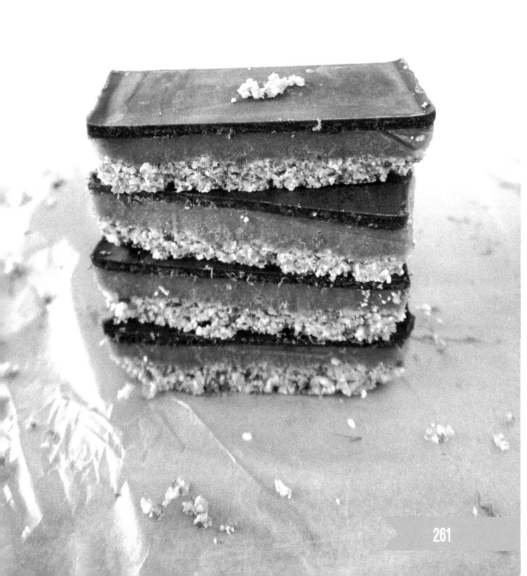

Caramello Cups

I use a mini cupcake tin and liners for this recipe, but you can choose any size and shape you'd like.

INGREDIENTS (MAKES 20)

For the Caramel
1/2 cup unhulled tahini
1/2 pure maple syrup or date paste
1/2 tsp vanilla
1/4 cup coconut butter OR coconut oil (melted)
Tiny pinch pink Himalayan salt

For the Chocolate
1 cup cacao butter
2 tbsp cacao powder
2 tbsp pure maple syrup
1/2 tsp vanilla powder or extract
1/2 tsp ground cinnamon (optional)

METHOD

Melt the cacao butter in a small saucepan or in a double boiler. Add remaining ingredients and stir until thick and velvety.

Spoon a layer of chocolate into the bottom of each cupcake liner. You only want to use half of the mix for this stage, as you will need the other half for the top layer. When finished, put the tray in the fridge and prepare the caramel.

Add all ingredients except for the coconut butter/oil to a bowl and mix until smooth. Add the coconut butter and mix until smooth and creamy.

Take the chocolate out of the fridge. It should now be firm. Spoon a layer of caramel (equal amounts) on top of each chocolate piece. Return to the fridge when finished.

When the caramel has somewhat set, spoon equal amounts of chocolate on top and return to the fridge to set. If the chocolate has started to thicken or harden, place back on the stove and heat gently.

VARIATION

For peanut butter cups, omit the coconut oil from the caramel and swap the tahini for peanut butter!

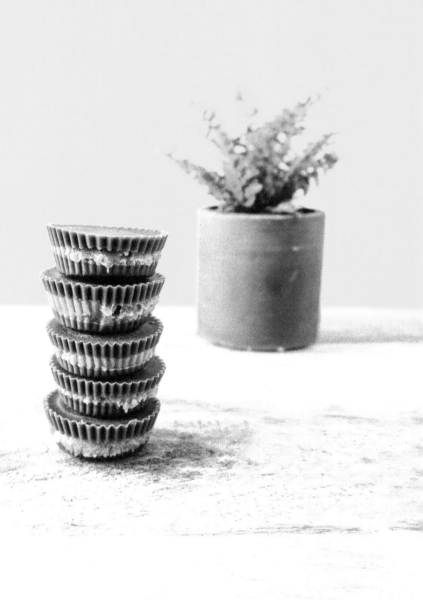

Caramel Twiks

These caramel twiks are a hit in my house and at our dinner parties. I prefer a more 'almondy' caramel, so I add 3.5tbsp of almond butter to the caramel, but if you prefer a 'datey' caramel, add 3 tbsp. You'll have to prepare the base and caramel ahead of time to allow it to freeze, before cutting it up and dipping it into chocolate.

INGREDIENTS (MAKES 12 LARGE STICKS)

For the Biscuit Base

1 cup cashews
1 cup macadamias
1 tbsp lucuma powder (optional)
2 tbsp pure maple syrup
Pinch pink Himalayan salt

For the Chocolate

1 cup cacao butter
2 tbsp cacao powder
2 tbsp pure maple syrup
1/2 tsp vanilla powder or extract
1/2 tsp ground cinnamon (optional)

For the Caramel

15 Medjool dates (pitted)
3 - 3.5 tbsp almond butter
2 tbsp coconut butter OR coconut oil (melted)
1 tsp vanilla powder
Tiny pinch pink Himalayan salt
4 - 6 tbsp filtered water, added gradually

METHOD

Add all biscuit base ingredients to a food processor or blender, and blitz until the mixture comes together and resembles a crumbly dough.

Press the dough into a medium-sized rectangular tray (I use a bread baking tin) lined with parchment paper and place in the freezer. Prepare the caramel.

Add all caramel ingredients except for the coconut oil/butter to a food processor, and pulse until smooth. Add the coconut oil/butter and pulse until combined. Spread over the biscuit base and freeze for at least 2 hours, then cut into long, equal-sized sticks.

Prepare the chocolate when the caramel and base are frozen, or solid enough to cut up without it falling apart.

Melt cacao butter in a small saucepan or in a double boiler. Add remaining ingredients and stir until thick and velvety.

Dip and coat each stick with chocolate and place on a plate lined with parchment paper. I find this step is easiest working with frozen sticks, as a thick layer of chocolate hardens and sets immediately. Otherwise, only a thin layer of chocolate will cover the stick, and you will have to dip the stick in chocolate again.

Store in the fridge in an airtight container for up to a week, or store in the freezer for up to 6 weeks. I prefer these stored in the freezer and either eaten straight away or eaten after 5 - 10 minutes out of the freezer.

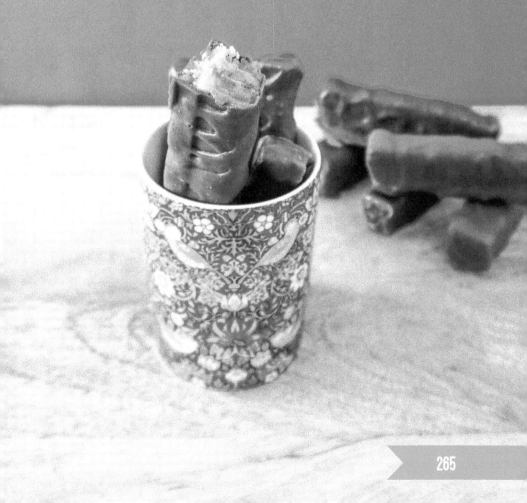

Pina Colada Cheezecake Jars

One of my absolute favourite combos is pineapple and coconut. Although, anything fruit is my favourite! These cheezecakes are raw and can be served in individual jars (which look super cool) or can be made in a lined cupcake tin for mini-cheezecakes, or made into one large cheezecake. To make this recipe less nut-heavy, you can also use fresh coconut meat combined with the coconut water to replace the cashews in the cheeze layer. Both variations are divine!

INGREDIENTS (MAKES ABOUT 12 MINI CHEESECAKES OR 6 JARS)

For the base
1 cup almonds/almond meal or cashews
1 cup shredded coconut
6 - 7 Medjool dates (pitted)
Tiny pinch pink Himalayan salt

For the Fruity Toppings
1/2 - 1 ripe pineapple

For the Coconut 'Cheeze' Layer
2 cups cashews (soaked in filtered water for at least 4 hours)
1/4 cup pure maple syrup
1/2 cup liquid (a mixture of juice from the pineapple or coconut milk, see below*)
1 tsp vanilla extract
Approximately 1/3 cup fresh lime juice
1/2 cup coconut butter or coconut oil (melted)
1/2 cup shredded coconut

METHOD

In a food processor, blitz all of the base ingredients until mixture sticks together and forms a dough. Add more dates if needed. Press into jars or a lined cupcake tray.

Prepare the pineapple. Remove the skin and the hard center, and chop into small pieces. Add about 2 cups of the pineapple to a food processor or blender to make crushed pineapple.

* Push some of the pineapple through a sieve to collect 1/2 cup juice. Otherwise use coconut milk or filtered water. This depends on whether you want a slightly pineapple-coconut tasting cheeze or purely coconut.

Blend all 'cheeze' ingredients together adding coconut butter/oil last. Only add coconut oil once the mixture is thick and smooth like cream. If the cheeze is too thick, gradually add more liquid until thick and creamy. Pour cream on to crusts and place in the fridge or freezer. Blending the cream tends to make the cream smoother than using a food processor. Use a blender or a stick blender for this step if you can.

Once set, sprinkle the top of the cheesecake with shredded coconut, and then top with the puréed pineapple. If the pineapple is too runny, drink some of the juice first. Add more pineapple purée if needed.

If not eating on the same day, store in the freezer until ready to eat. Storing in the freezer will reduce the chance of the base becoming soggy. Allow to thaw for 30 minutes before serving.

VARIATIONS

Replace the pineapple with fresh puréed strawberries or raspberries, and a dash of pure maple syrup and lime juice. Yum!

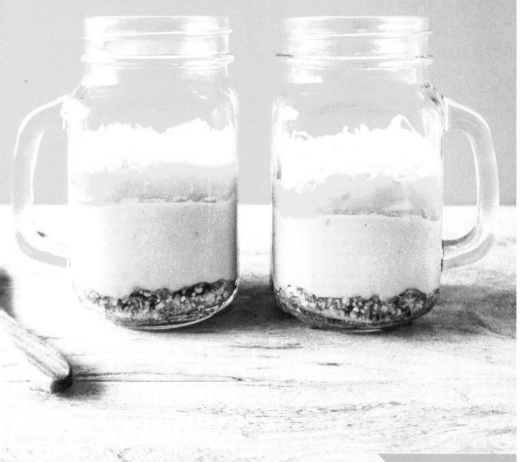

Mini Mango and Passionfruit Cheezecakes

These cheezecakes are my other favourite combo: mango and passionfruit! This recipe is my all-time-favourite dessert.

INGREDIENTS (MAKES ABOUT 12 MINI CHEESECAKES OR 6 JARS)

For the base
1 cup almonds or cashews
1 cup shredded coconut
6 - 7 Medjool dates (pitted)
Tiny pinch pink Himalayan salt

For the Fruity Toppings
2 ripe mangoes
Approximately 10 - 12 ripe passionfruit

For the 'Cheeze' Layer
2 cups cashews (soaked in filtered water for at least 4 hours)
1/4 cup pure maple syrup
1/2 cup filtered water
1 tsp vanilla extract
Approximately 1/3 cup fresh lime juice
1/2 cup coconut butter or coconut oil (melted)

METHOD

Process all of the base ingredients until mixture sticks together and forms a dough. Add more dates if needed. Press into jars or lined cupcake tray.

Blend all 'cheeze' ingredients together adding coconut butter/oil last. Only add coconut butter/oil once the mixture is smooth, like cream. Pour cream on to crusts and place in the fridge or freezer.

Peel and purée the mangoes, scoop out the passionfruit pulp, and add to a small bowl. If the passionfruit are on the sour side, stir in a few drops of pure maple syrup before adding to the mango purée. Mix well. Evenly pour fruit on top of cheezecakes. The trick here is to pour a thick layer of fruit purée, so it bursts with flavour!

If not eating on the same day these are prepared, store in the freezer until ready to eat. You can add the purée to the top of the cheezecakes before storing in the freezer or add the fresh purée just before eating. Storing in the freezer will reduce the chance of the base becoming soggy. Allow to thaw for 10 minutes before serving.

VARIATIONS

Replace the mango and passionfruit with fresh puréed pink pitaya/ dragonfruit, or raspberries. Yum!

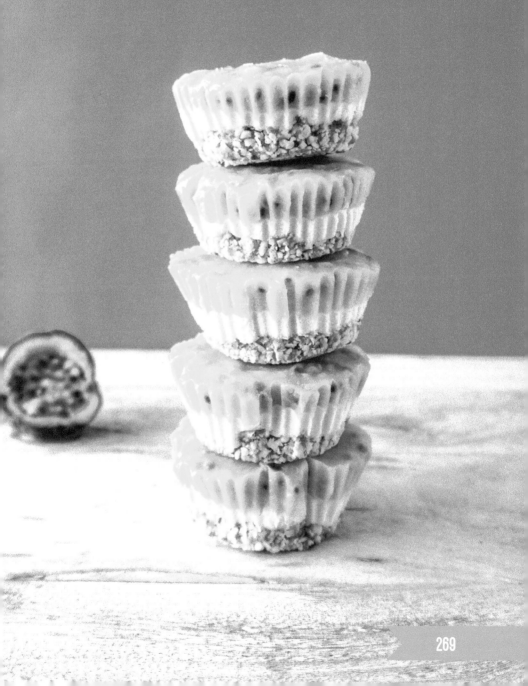

Neopolitan Nicecream

An old pre-vegan and childhood favourite, remade!

INGREDIENTS (SERVES 3)

9 frozen bananas
1 tsp vanilla powder or extract
1/2 - 1 cup plant-milk

For the strawberry flavour

2 cups frozen strawberries
Dash lemon juice
Dash pure maple syrup

For the chocolate flavour

3 - 4 tsp cacao powder
Dash pure maple syrup
1/2 tsp ground cinnamon

METHOD

Add bananas, milk, and vanilla to a blender and blitz until smooth and creamy. Quickly separate the mixture into 3 different bowls. Keep in the freezer until ready.

Add one part back to the blender and blitz with the frozen strawberries, lemon juice and maple syrup. Put back in the freezer.

Blitz another part of the banana mixture with the cacao, maple syrup, and cinnamon. Put back in the freezer.

When you're ready to serve, scoop each flavour into 3 bowls and top with chopped chocolate. I use raw mylk chocolate or chopped strawberries.

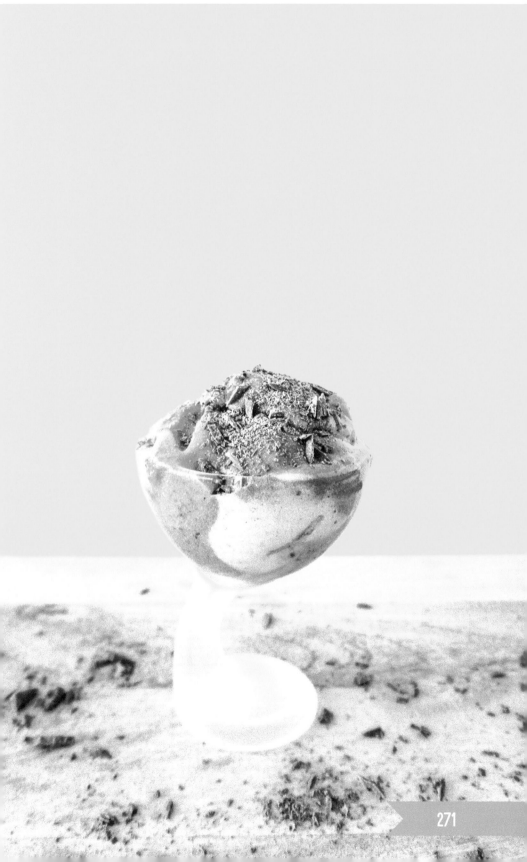

No-Churn Berry Coconut Nicecream

If you have an ice cream maker, feel free to use it!

INGREDIENTS (SERVES 4 - 6)

4 cups frozen strawberries or mixed berries
2 x 15 oz/400ml cans coconut cream (BPA-free)
1 tsp vanilla extract or seeds from 1 vanilla pod
1/2 cup pure maple syrup
1 - 2 tsp fresh lemon juice

METHOD

Scoop the thick coconut cream out of the can and add to a bowl. Whip with an electric beater until thick and creamy and soft peaks form. It's important to get to the soft-peak stage so the nicecream will set creamy, rather than icy. If the cream won't whip, place in the fridge for 20 minutes and try again. Set aside. Add remaining ingredients to a blender and blitz until smooth and creamy. Fold into whipped coconut cream and mix until combined.

Pour mixture into a freezer-safe tray and place in the freezer and cover. Gently whisk mixture every 20 minutes for the next 3 hours. Every time you whisk it, it should become thicker. Make sure to scrape down the sides if the nicecream is setting.

Once thick enough to scoop, serve immediately, or store in the freezer until needed. Thaw for 10 minutes before eating and eat within 2 weeks.

TIP

Scoop only the coconut cream, leaving the coconut water behind. Use the leftover water in a smoothie or other recipe.

VARIATIONS

Leave out the strawberries for a nice coconut vanilla flavour. Or replace the strawberries with 3 tbsp cacao powder and make a batch of Choctella Sauce (see page 196) to top. Yum!

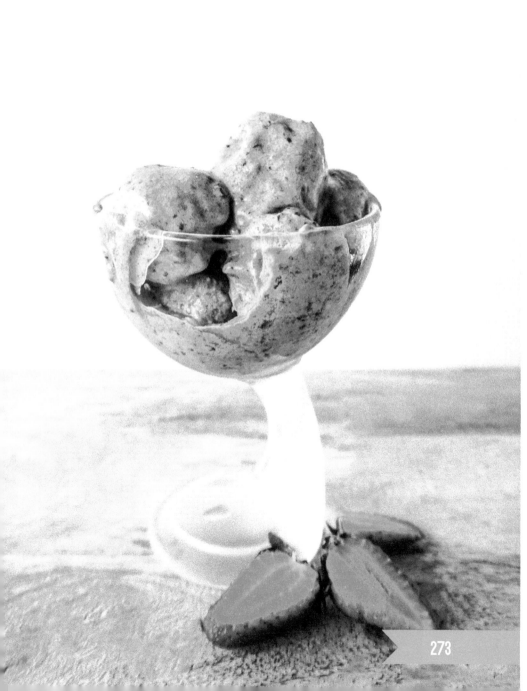

Snickerz Nicecream

A decadent take on the simple nicecream!

INGREDIENTS (SERVES 2 - 3)

6 - 8 frozen bananas
2 tbsp mesquite powder
1/2 tsp vanilla extract
1/2 cup plant-milk
Raw chocolate (see page 260) OR Choctella Sauce (see page 196)
Raw caramel sauce (see page 260)
1/2 cup peanuts (chopped)

METHOD

Make the chocolate and caramel first.

Add bananas, mesquite, vanilla, and plant-milk to a blender and blitz until smooth and creamy. Using a spoon, take a spoonful of chocolate sauce and line the inside of the jars or glasses. Scoop some of the banana nicecream into the jars, then top with caramel sauce, peanuts, and chocolate. Repeat.

Finish with chocolate sauce and chopped peanuts. Devour straight away.

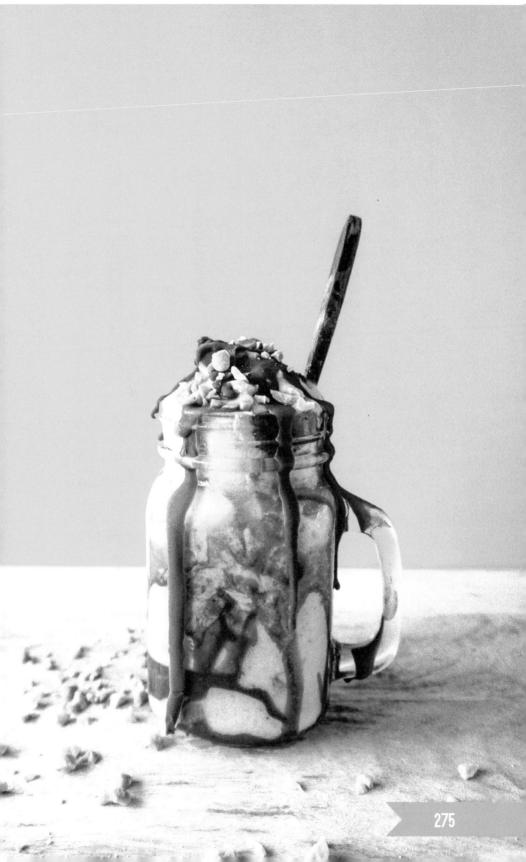

Apple, Rhubarb and Mixed Berry Crumble

I love crumble in the cooler months. All sorts of crumble! I often bake this without apples too! Granny Smiths work best but any apples will do. I use frozen mixed berries because I dislike cooking fresh berries, as I prefer to eat them as is! But you can use either. I also prefer to use a shallow dish because I like a similar crumble-to-fruit ratio. Double the fruit if you'd prefer more filling. To make this nut-free, use a blend of buckwheat flour and rolled oats.

INGREDIENTS (SERVES 5)

Fruit Filling

1 apple (thinly sliced or diced, peeled)
2 cups of mixed berries
(strawberries halved or quartered)
2 stalks of rhubarb (sliced
into 3cm pieces)
2 tbsp date syrup, pure maple
syrup or coconut sugar
2 tsp tapioca or arrowroot
flour/starch
2 tsp lemon juice (optional)

Crumble

1 cup rolled oats (can
use buckwheat flour)
1 cup chopped cashews, or chopped
macadamias, or almond meal
1/2 cup shredded coconut
1/2 cup coconut sugar
3 - 4 tbsp coconut oil (melted)
2 Medjool dates (pitted)
1/2 - 1 tsp ground cinnamon (optional)
Slivered almonds to top (optional)

METHOD

Preheat oven to 190C/374F. Place apples, berries and rhubarb into an ovenproof dish, top with sweetener and tapioca. Mix thoroughly. Bake fruit for about 15 minutes.

While the fruit is baking, add all crumble ingredients to a food processor and gently blitz, leaving some texture. The crumble should resemble a crumbly dough. If the mixture is still dry and hasn't come together, add more coconut oil or another date. Adjust as required.

Take the fruit out of the oven and evenly spread the crumble on top of the fruit filling. Sprinkle slivered almonds over the top if you prefer. Bake for approximately 15 minutes or until the crumble is golden and the fruit is bubbling around the edges. Try not to overcook the fruit.

Keep an eye on the crumble and make sure the top doesn't burn.

I bake this dish in two parts because the baking times vary. The rhubarb takes a little longer to cook than the crumble, and rhubarb must be cooked properly. You can bake both sections together, however, be mindful that the crumble may begin to burn before the rhubarb has cooked through.

Serve with vanilla nicecream or Cashew Cream (see page 214)

VARIATIONS

Replace the rhubarb with 2 - 3 pears and/or peaches. Yum!

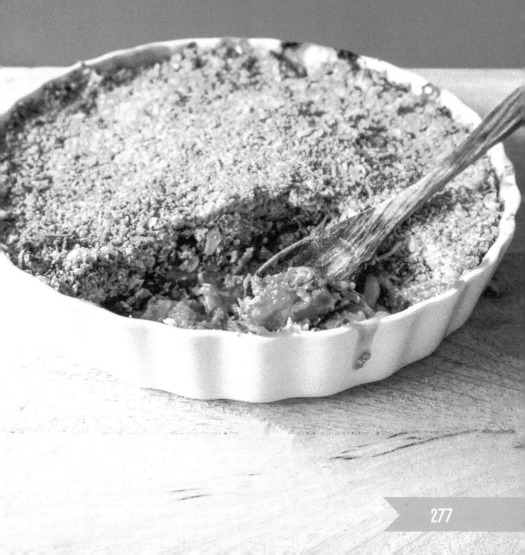

Chocolate Cremestons

These biscuits are inspired by an old pre-vegan favourite, Kingstons. You can make these completely raw, or add the biscuits to a dehydrator, or bake them to give them a nice crunch.

INGREDIENTS (MAKES 8 LARGE COOKIES OR 12 SMALLER COOKIES)

Cookie Dough

1 cup cashews
1 cup shredded coconut
7 Medjool dates (pitted)
Pinch pink Himalayan salt

Chocolate Creme

1/2 cup coconut butter or coconut oil (semi-soft, not liquefied)
2 tbsp cacao powder
2 tbsp pure maple syrup
1/2 tsp vanilla extract
1/2 tsp ground cinnamon
Small pinch pink Himalayan salt

METHOD

In a food processor or powerful blender, pulse all of the biscuit ingredients together until you get a semi-sticky dough texture. Spoon out a spoonful at a time and roll into small balls, then flatten the balls into discs. Do this with the entire batch and place on a tray lined with parchment paper and put in the fridge. If you want a crunchy texture, place in a dehydrator for a few hours, or bake at 160C/320F for 5 - 10 minutes (keep an eye on them). If you bake the cookies, the cookies will be soft once removed from the oven, but they will harden slightly once cooled.

Blend or process all of the chocolate crème ingredients until you get a thick, creamy, frosting-like texture. I find this step is easiest to make using a stick blender and beaker. If the cream becomes too runny, place in the fridge for a short time and blend again. This process works best when the oil is soft but not liquefied.

Remove the cookies from the fridge or oven (and allow to cool). Place a small spoonful of chocolate crème on top of one cookie and place another cookie on top, so the crème is sandwiched in the middle. If the crème is too soft, place the cookies in the fridge for 5 or so minutes before adding the top cookie. Repeat till finished and place in the fridge and allow to set. Store in an airtight container for up to 2 weeks.

TIP

This chocolate crème recipe doubles as chocolate frosting, so use this recipe next time you need to frost a cake or cupcakes. Yum!

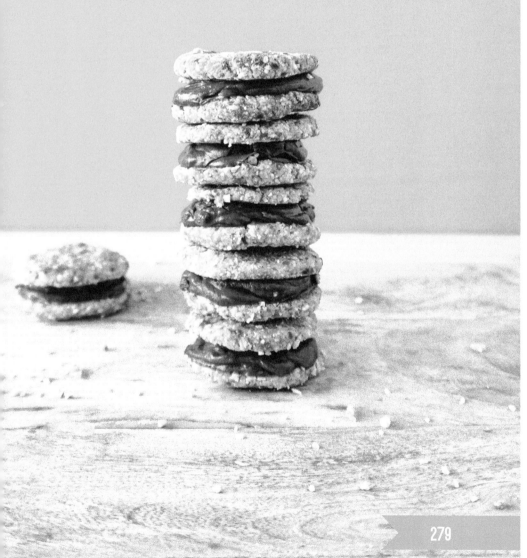

Banana, Choc Chip & Peanut Butter Muffins

These are my family's favourite muffins. I'm not a huge fan of peanut butter, but peanut butter fans tend to like these. For gluten-free baking, I generally use buckwheat flour and chickpea flour (besan flour) mixed with tapioca/arrowroot flour or flax eggs. Adding tapioca or flax eggs helps to bind and lighten the mixture. I also don't like to add xanthum gum or guar gum, and tapioca flour and flax eggs help to replace the gums. Using banana in baking gives it a nice, mellow banana flavour and can also replace the eggs and oil, keeping the muffins moist. The following muffins are completely oil-free!

INGREDIENTS
(MAKES 12 CUPCAKES)

3/4 cup mashed bananas
(about 2 medium bananas)
2 flax eggs (2 tbsp flaxmeal
+ 4 tbsp filtered water)
2 tbsp pure maple syrup
3 tbsp plant-milk

1 tbsp vanilla extract
1.5 tsp apple cider vinegar
1.5 cups buckwheat flour
(can use besan flour)
1 tsp baking soda
1 tsp ground cinnamon
Small pinch Pink Himalayan salt
1/4 - 1/2 cup dark chocolate
chips (or chopped chocolate)
Smooth peanut butter

METHOD

Preheat oven to 180C/356F and line muffin tray with cupcake cases.

To a medium bowl, add all dry ingredients, except for the chocolate chips, and mix well, sifting flour and baking soda.

To a large bowl, add the wet ingredients, except for the peanut butter, and mix well, then add dry ingredients to wet ingredients and mix. The consistency should be thick but runny, like cooked oatmeal. Adjust milk or flour quantities if you need to. Fold in chocolate chips.

Divide evenly between the cupcake cases, only filling each case half way. Using a teaspoon, carefully spoon 1 teaspoon of peanut butter into each casing, swirl the peanut butter, so it becomes part of the batter. Top with the remaining batter and swirl the muffin again. An easier alternative is to spoon the peanut butter on to the top of each muffin making sure to swirl the peanut butter, so it becomes part of the batter. You can also use a cupcake corer and add the peanut butter after the muffins are ready.

Bake for about 15 minutes or until a skewer or knife comes out clean. If you find your oven is cooking the tops too fast, drop the oven temperature down to 170C/338F until cooked. Leave muffins to cool in the tray for 10 minutes, then transfer the muffins to a wire rack cooler to cool completely.

VARIATIONS

Make banana coconut muffins by replacing the peanut butter and chocolate chips with 1 cup of shredded coconut. Omit the peanut butter for banana chocolate chip, or add 1 cup of fresh or frozen raspberries and 1 cup of shredded coconut for raspberry coconut muffins. Yum!

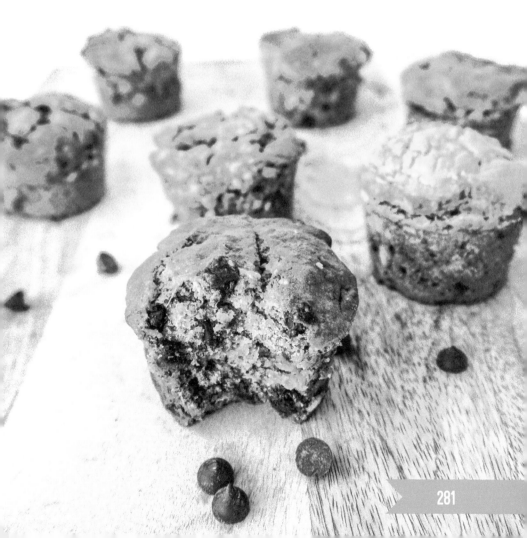

Sticky Date Muffins

These muffins are my favourite. A healthy snack that also doubles as a dessert!

INGREDIENTS (MAKES 12)

1.5 cups buckwheat flour (can use besan flour)
3/4 cup coconut sugar
1 tsp baking soda
1 tsp ground cinnamon
Small pinch Pink Himalayan salt
3/4 cup puréed bananas (about 2 medium bananas)
2 flax eggs (2 tbsp flaxmeal + 4 tbsp filtered water)
1/2 cup plant-milk
1 tbsp vanilla extract
1.5 tsp apple cider vinegar
1/2 cup Medjool dates (chopped) + 4 to garnish

METHOD

Preheat oven to 180C/356F and line muffin tray with cupcake cases.

Sift dry ingredients in a medium bowl and mix well. The coconut sugar won't fit through the sieve so just tip it into the bowl.

To a separate large bowl, add the wet ingredients, except for the dates, and mix well. Add the dry ingredients to the wet ingredients and combine. The consistency should be thick and sticky but runny, like cooked oatmeal. Adjust milk or flour quantities if you need to. Fold in chopped dates.

Divide evenly between the 12 cases and add 1/4 of a date to the top of each muffin.

Bake for about 15 minutes or until a skewer or knife comes out clean. Leave muffins to cool in the tray for 10 minutes, then transfer to a wire rack cooler to cool completely.

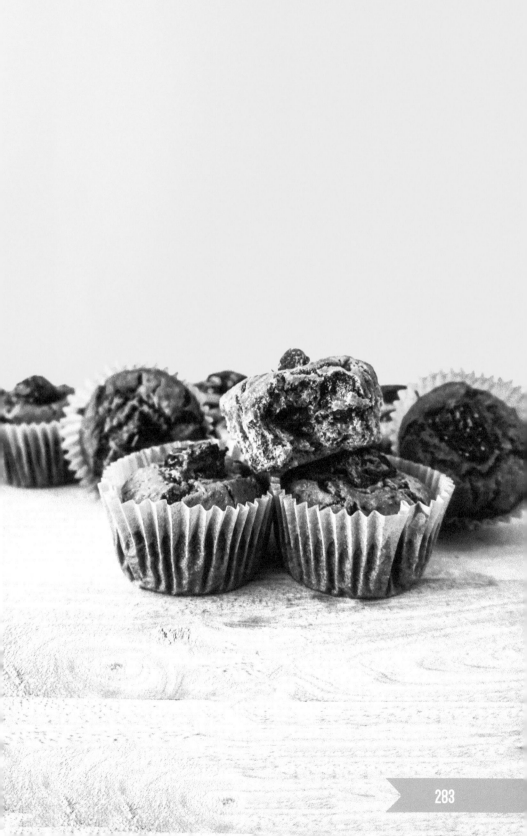

Choc Mint Cupcakes

I love the simplicity of a choc-mint ganache to flavour these cupcakes!

INGREDIENTS (MAKES 12 CUPCAKES)

3/4 cup puréed bananas
(about 2 medium bananas)
2 flax eggs (2 tbsp flax meal
+ 4 tbsp filtered water)
1/2 cup pure maple syrup
1/2 cup to 3/4 plant-milk
1 tbsp vanilla extract
1.5 tsp apple cider vinegar
1.5 cups buckwheat flour
1/3 cup cacao powder

1/2 cup shredded coconut (optional)
1 tsp baking soda
1 tsp ground cinnamon
Small pinch Pink Himalayan salt

GANACHE

Preferred raw mint chocolate
Plant-milk
Dash of pure maple syrup (if needed)

METHOD

Preheat oven to 180C/356F and line cupcake tray with cupcake cases.

Add all dry ingredients to a medium bowl and mix well, sifting the flour and baking soda.

To a large bowl, add the wet ingredients and mix well. Add dry ingredients to the wet ingredients and mix. The consistency should be thick but runny, like cooked oatmeal. Adjust milk or flour quantities if you need to.

Divide the batter between the cupcake cases. Bake for about 15 minutes or until a skewer or knife comes out clean. If you find your oven is cooking the tops too fast, drop the oven temperature down to 170C/338F until cooked. Leave cupcakes to cool in the tray for 10 minutes, then transfer to a wire rack cooler to cool completely.

For the ganache, in a saucepan on a very low heat or a double boiler, melt a block of your preferred raw mint chocolate and gradually add milk until you have a thick sauce. Milk quantity will depend on how much chocolate you are melting, but it shouldn't be more than 1/2 cup. Allow to cool and use a knife or a piping bag to cover the tops of the cupcakes. If the ganache is too runny, place in the fridge until it thickens.

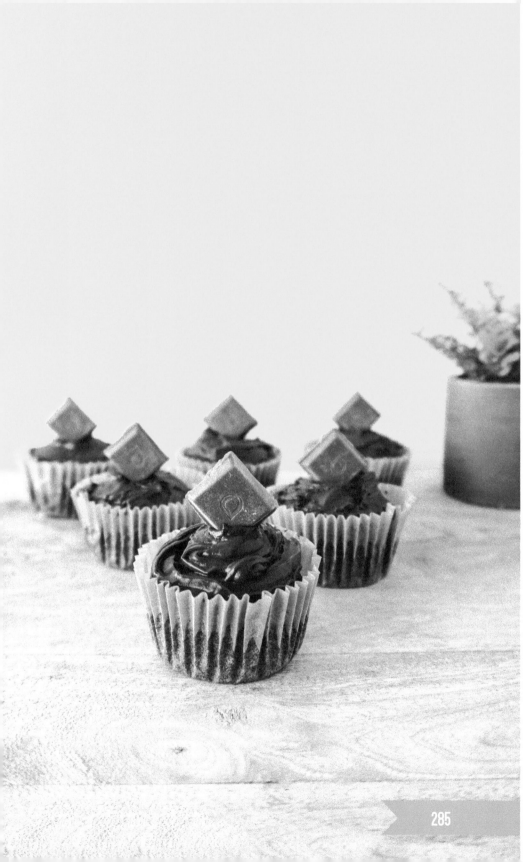

Chewy Chocolate Brownies

I've always preferred brownies with a bit of crunch and chewiness, but to make that happen the recipe must use sugar. And while these brownies still contain nutrients from the nuts, this recipe is more of a treat.

INGREDIENTS (MAKES 8 - 10 BROWNIES)

1 cup almond butter
1/2 cup coconut sugar
2 tbsp pure maple syrup or date syrup
5 tbsp cacao powder
1 tsp vanilla powder or extract
1/2 tsp ground cinnamon
1/2 tsp baking soda
Pinch pink Himalayan salt
1 flax egg (1 tbsp flax meal + 2 tbsp water)
1/2 cup peanuts, macadamias or almonds (halved)

METHOD

Preheat oven to 175C/350F. Make the flax egg and leave to the side. Combine the rest of the ingredients in a medium-sized bowl and mix until a soft dough forms. Remember to add the flax egg.

Press into a small, parchment-lined baking dish. The mixture should be thick, so you will need to use your hands to press the batter into the tray. Bake for about 20 minutes.

Allow to cool in the tray, and then cool completely on a wire rack before slicing it up. Store in the fridge in an airtight container for up to a week.

VARIATIONS

Replace the nuts with dark chocolate chunks or add a creamy ganache to the top for an extra treat (melted chocolate + dash of plant-milk). Eat as is or serve with vanilla nicecream. Yum!

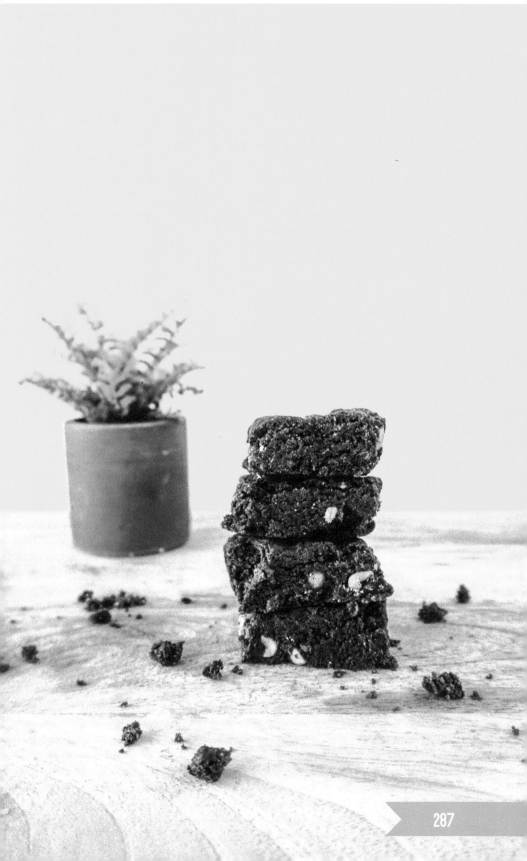

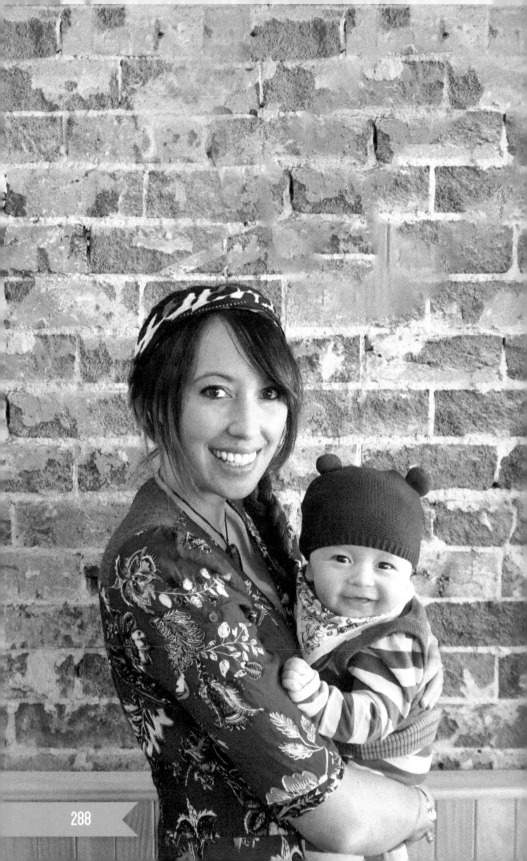

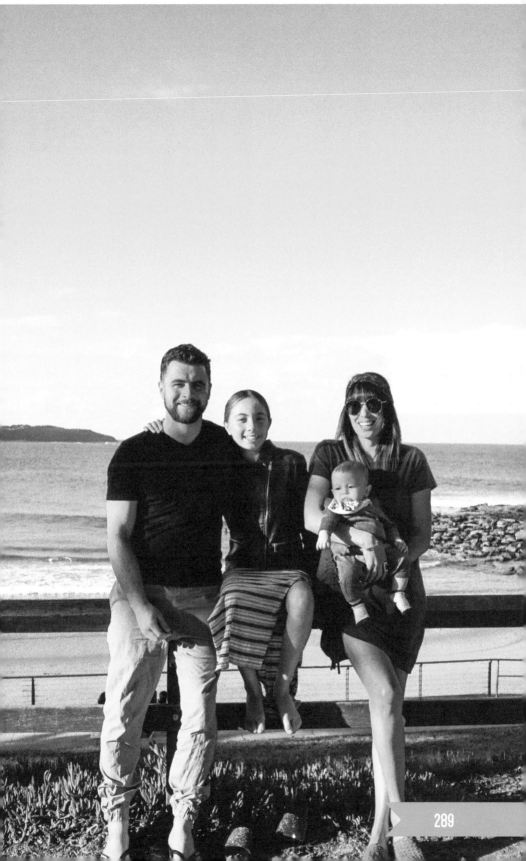

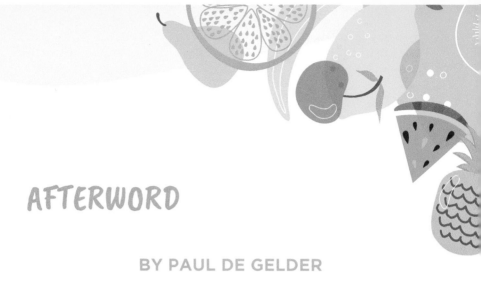

AFTERWORD

BY PAUL DE GELDER

From the moment in 2016 when I decided to leave meat and dairy behind I felt goodness in my soul.

Sure, the first time I tried to go plant-based I failed dismally within three days, but the seed had been planted and the Universe kept nudging me. It got to the point where it could no longer be ignored, and I truly believe that when the Universe seeks your attention you'd best prick up your ears lest you reap the consequences.

Even though I had become lactose intolerant at 15, I still had a healthy addiction to ice cream. Since there are plenty of other options now, that was the easy choice for the first food to go. Then I stopped eating red meat; no more kangaroo tacos or fillets in red wine jus. But, I was adamant.

I worked in the conservation realm trying to protect the animals, yet here I was eating them. That made me something that I hated: a hypocrite. It was high time that my ideals and my actions aligned, so, goodbye chicken. I was terrified. How will I get muscles without the bodybuilding staple of 'boobs from a chicken?' Chicken breast! I rarely steer away from a challenge and it wasn't like I was cutting off my *other* leg. I thought, if this doesn't work, I could always go back. The last vestige of animal exploitation and cruelty was on the chopping block: eggs.

Finally, I was plant-based and there was no turning back.

By taking this step I did something that I could never have foretold, I set a precedent. I became an example that others could follow, but with that came responsibility, so, I had to do it right.

It started with a little research, calculating how much of each nutrient I needed, especially protein, in order to eat this way and function at a higher physical level than most of the people around me. Only later did I realise how little I had to fear. By cutting out animal products, I was forced to eat more natural foods. I started with the basics, broccoli, carrots, and potatoes, and then added just about the whole produce section. My body thanked me for it. I haven't had a significant injury from training since the day I switched to a plant-based diet. That still blows my mind. I very rarely get sick, and if I do, the duration is shorter and far less severe than those around me. My fitness and lifestyle are uninterrupted, and I can focus on and achieve my goals, without the distractions and speed bumps of illness and injury. In one fell swoop, I no longer took in fungicides, pesticides, antibiotics, unnatural hormones, and the adrenaline, pain, and fear of animals.

We *are* what we eat, so why would you willingly add any of that to your life? And funnily enough, most people feel like it's the plant-based eaters that are extreme. Well, then let us be extreme.

Extreme in our compassion. Extreme in our lust for a healthy, disease-free life. Extreme in our love for our families and friends. Extreme in our passion to make a positive change in our world and in our bodies.

 I will never have to give birth and I count my blessings for that; I believe that I would die! Women are the creators, the mothers, the nurturers, and what you put into your body while you are pregnant nourishes, fuels, and moulds the health of your growing child. So, why wouldn't you choose the absolute best you can?

Candy, like myself, does not want to see people or animals suffer needlessly. We only wish to share the knowledge of how much better life can be, for us all. And this book is a prime example of sharing such knowledge.

Enjoy the ride; it's really quite amazing to show the world what is possible when you break down those old beliefs about healthy eating and shift into a higher gear with plants.

PAUL DE GELDER

(Author, Motivational Speaker, Navy Diver, Shark Attack Survivor, Conservationist)

www.pauldegelder.com

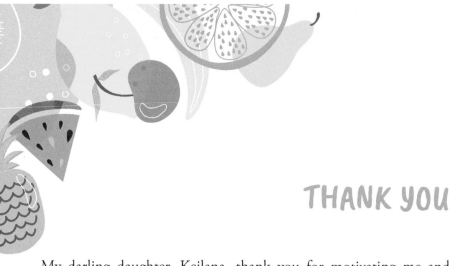

THANK YOU

My darling daughter, Keilana, thank you for motivating me and helping me make and perfect the recipes in this book. Without your help, I'd still be in the kitchen trying to finalize everything. There were plenty of times when my pregnant-third-trimester-body didn't want to spend yet another day in the kitchen, and you helped me every step of the way. You truly inspire me, and you made me so proud by seeing your creativeness soar. You are a natural in the kitchen and your attention to detail is astounding. Thank you for always eagerly helping and supporting me. I love seeing how compassionate you are; when you save bugs from drowning in the swimming pool, when you move caterpillars off of the footpath, or when you pick up litter at the beach, your kind and caring soul is exactly what the world needs.

Kaimana, my content, happy, chilled-out, cheeky baby boy, thank you for inspiring this book and for helping me understand just how connected mamas truly are to our babies. I never knew that anything was missing in my life until you came along. I count my lucky stars to have your peaceful presence and brightness around me. For someone so small, you're so full of love. My heart is so full!

Mike, thank you for your patience, for not complaining when you came home from work and I was still focused on this book; for your help with the photography, and for not looking at our weekly grocery bill while I was baking up a storm! Thank you for eating every successful and unsuccessful recipe attempt without batting an eyelid – you know how much I dislike wasting food, and I thank you for your incredible support. And thank you for trusting me and believing in me when I wanted us to go vegan.

Suzy Amis Cameron, thank you so much for being part of this book. I can't begin to describe how excited I was when you accepted my invitation to write the foreword. I've followed your journey for a few years and I've seen how much you've done for animals, the planet, and our fellow human beings. I can't wait to read your book, OMD! Thank you so much!

Damien Mander, I can't even begin to explain how much you inspire and motivate me. The conservation and humanitarian work that you do is beyond incredible, and I am so humbled and proud to know you, and to have you as part of this book. I love your humility and how quick you are to support and compliment others, without realizing that you do far more than many of us, combined! You really do give so much more love than you take! Your leadership and passion for all life is contagious and I have so much respect for you. Thank you for all that you do.

Paul De Gelder, your optimism and light are infectious, and I'm so honoured to have you as part of this book. Thank you for taking the time to write the powerful afterword, for helping our animal counterparts, and inspiring others to follow a compassionate lifestyle.

To my family and friends who have encouraged me to write a cookbook over the past few years, thank you for planting that seed. That seed finally grew!

I would like to thank Ethical Press Publishers and Richell Balansag for helping make this manuscript become a literary cookbook! And many thanks to Tania Niwa for delivering such a beautiful cover photo.

Thank you to my social media family, for your kind and loving words, and for supporting this book long before it was released. I can't tell you how happy I was when you subscribed to the website, when you wrote messages of encouragement, and when I received your emails. This book has become a reality because of your support. Thank you!

Lastly, to all of my fellow animal-loving, Earth-adoring, plant-eaters: thank you for being the change you wish to see in the world!

CM xxxx

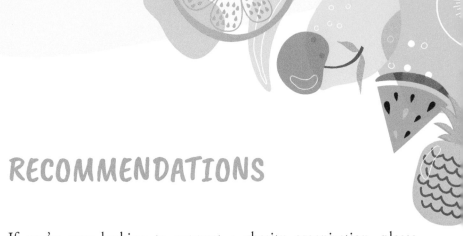

RECOMMENDATIONS

If you're ever looking to support a charity organization, please consider supporting your local animal sanctuaries, or your local conservation, humanitarian, and rescue groups. Or please support the amazing work of the charities below.

International Anti-Poaching Foundation www.iapf.org

Rainforest Rescue www.rainforestrescue.org.au

Reach Out World Wide www.roww.org

Sea Shepherd www.seashepherd.org

Shelter Ugolyok www.instagram.com/shelter_ugolyok

WIRES Wildlife Rescue www.wires.org.au

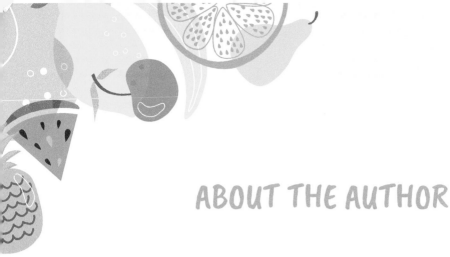

ABOUT THE AUTHOR

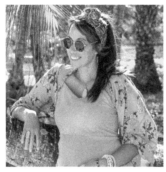

Candy Marx is a Registered Plant-based Nutritionist, Registered Master Herbalist, Social Entrepreneur, Conservationist, Writer, Intuition Mentor, a Mama of two, and a Kind Living and Wellness Influencer behind the popular Instagram account and website, Plantfed Mama.

An award-winning ex-fashion footwear designer, Candy left high-end fashion and changed direction after discovering how detrimental leather is to animals and the planet. Leather is listed twice on the World's Top Ten Pollutants from factory farms and leather tanneries. Rebranding to **KSKYE the Label**, the eco-vegan social brand supports artisans from developing countries, and several animal welfare, conservation and humanitarian charities by donating 100% of the profits from its BE KIND Series.

Also the founder of the **Plantfed Mama Herb Shop**, Candy is passionate about plant-based eating, holistic health and wellness, spirituality, humanity, and being kind to all life. Originally from Hawkes Bay, New Zealand, Candy currently lives with her vegan family in Sydney, Australia.